T0172743

The Immunology of
Human Reproduction

The Immunology of Human Reproduction

Isaac T Manyonda PhD MRCOG

Department of Obstetrics and Gynaecology
St George's Hospital Medical School
London, UK

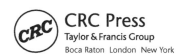

CRC Press
Taylor & Francis Group
Boca Raton London New York

CRC Press is an imprint of the
Taylor & Francis Group, an **informa** business
A TAYLOR & FRANCIS BOOK

CRC Press
Taylor & Francis Group
6000 Broken Sound Parkway NW, Suite 300
Boca Raton, FL 33487-2742

First issued in paperback 2019

© 2006 by Taylor & Francis Group, LLC
CRC Press is an imprint of Taylor & Francis Group, an Informa business

No claim to original U.S. Government works

ISBN-13: 978-1-85070-791-2 (hbk)
ISBN-13: 978-0-367-39123-2 (pbk)

This book contains information obtained from authentic and highly regarded sources. Reasonable efforts have been made to publish reliable data and information, but the author and publisher cannot assume responsibility for the validity of all materials or the consequences of their use. The authors and publishers have attempted to trace the copyright holders of all material reproduced in this publication and apologize to copyright holders if permission to publish in this form has not been obtained. If any copyright material has not been acknowledged please write and let us know so we may rectify in any future reprint.

Except as permitted under U.S. Copyright Law, no part of this book may be reprinted, reproduced, transmitted, or utilized in any form by any electronic, mechanical, or other means, now known or hereafter invented, including photocopying, microfilming, and recording, or in any information storage or retrieval system, without written permission from the publishers.

For permission to photocopy or use material electronically from this work, please access www. copyright.com (http://www.copyright.com/) or contact the Copyright Clearance Center, Inc. (CCC), 222 Rosewood Drive, Danvers, MA 01923, 978-750-8400. CCC is a not-for-profit organization that provides licenses and registration for a variety of users. For organizations that have been granted a photocopy license by the CCC, a separate system of payment has been arranged.

Trademark Notice: Product or corporate names may be trademarks or registered trademarks, and are used only for identification and explanation without intent to infringe.

British Library Cataloguing in Publication Data
Data available on application

Library of Congress Cataloging-in-Publication Data
Data available on application

Composition by Parthenon Publishing

Visit the Taylor & Francis Web site at
http://www.taylorandfrancis.com

and the CRC Press Web site at
http://www.crcpress.com

Contents

Preface

The main function of the immune system is to defend the body against invasion by bacteria, viruses and other pathogenic organisms. The immune system is also thought to mount surveillance against malignancy. In other words, pathogens and malignant cells are 'foreign' or 'non-self', and, therefore, the fundamental function of the immune system is to recognize and eliminate 'non-self'. This fundamental function raises a major issue with regard to human pregnancy: the human fetus, which is essentially 'non-self' as it derives half its genetic information from the father, is not treated as 'non-self' and eliminated, but in fact is welcomed, nourished for 9 months and then nurtured for the next 18 years! Why the fetus is not eliminated by the immune system of the mother has puzzled and fascinated biologists for years, and has given rise to the subject of reproductive immunology. The paradox became acutely apparent in the late 1940s/early 1950s following discovery of the laws of transplantation immunology by Peter Medawar and his colleagues. Medawar himself, probably one of the greatest immunologists as well as a philosopher, crystallized the paradox in these words: 'The immunological problem of pregnancy may be formulated thus: How does the pregnant mother contrive to nourish within itself, for many months or weeks, a fetus that is an antigenically foreign body?'

Many have speculated on the wide-ranging benefits that might accrue from the unraveling of the mechanisms by which the fetus eludes the maternal immune system. Rational strategies might evolve for the treatment of diseases of pregnancy thought to have an immunological basis (e.g. recurrent spontaneous miscarriage, pre-eclampsia and intrauterine growth restriction); organ transplantation programs might benefit by emulating nature's strategies in creating a perfect allograft; clues might emerge as to how tumors escape immunosurveillance, and new treatments might therefore be developed.

Peter Medawar's thinking on this matter has dominated ideas on the maternal–fetal immunological relationship to this day. Medawar himself conducted no research to try to resolve the paradox, but suggested that the placenta must play a central role in fetal survival, as the trophoblast cells interface with the mother. However, his other proposals – maternal immunosuppression and immaturity of fetal antigens – together with subsequent diverse hypotheses by others have not withstood the test of time. Probably central to the failure to arrive at a conclusive resolution of this paradox is the fact that the fetus should really not be considered an allograft in the conventional sense. While the adaptive immune response would be central to conventional concepts of the rejection of an allograft, recent research in reproductive immunology would suggest that the innate immune system might, in fact, play a more important role in the maternal–fetal immunological relationship. These and other issues are explored in this book, which is aimed at readers, predominantly obstetricians and gynecologists, who are often daunted by the subject of immunology, yet wish to gain a better understanding of the subject. It is not intended as a detailed exposé on immunology, nor does it intend to deal with state-of-the-art research in the field of reproductive immunology. Rather, the aim is to equip the reader with sufficient knowledge of immunological concepts to allow an understanding of the current thinking and approaches to reproductive immunology. Further reading is suggested where appropriate.

A guide to cell types

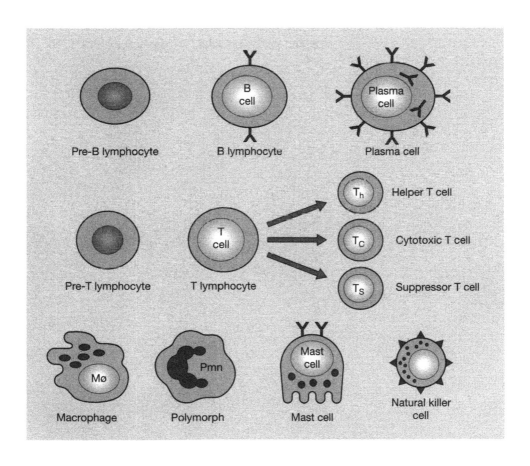

1

Essential concepts in basic immunology

The human body has three lines of defense against invasion by external pathogens, namely:

- The physical barrier – first line

- The innate immune system – second line

- The adaptive immune system – third line

THE PHYSICAL BARRIER

Although it is often forgotten, in fact the *physical barrier* plays a critical role in the defense against infection, and indeed without its contribution it is highly unlikely that the innate and adaptive immune systems could cope. The physical barrier comprises an extensive surface area that includes the skin, covering approximately $2\,m^2$ in the adult, and mucous membranes that line the digestive, reproductive and respiratory systems, measuring approximately $400\,m^2$.

INNATE VERSUS ADAPTIVE IMMUNE SYSTEM

It is customary to divide the immune system into 'innate' and 'adaptive' components. The *innate immune system* is described as consisting of the following constituents:

(1) Soluble elements, including complement, acute phase proteins and interferon;

(2) Professional phagocytes, including macrophages and neutrophils;

(3) Natural killer cells.

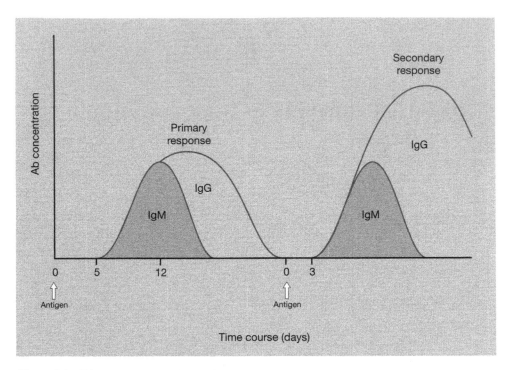

Figure 1.1 Primary and secondary antibody responses. Ab, antibody; Ig, immunoglobulin

The essential characteristic of the innate immune system is that the response to any given pathogen is not affected by previous exposure, and remains of the same magnitude each time the system is challenged by pathogens. The *adaptive immune system*, which comprises T and B lymphocytes, antibodies, receptors, etc., has four fundamental features, namely *memory*, *specificity*, *diversity* and *tolerance* to 'self'. *Memory* is demonstrated by the fact that the human species rarely suffers twice from certain infections (e.g. chicken-pox): the first contact with an infectious agent imparts memory, so that subsequent infection is repelled. This introduces the concept of *primary and secondary* immune responses: the primary response occurs on first contact with a pathogen, and is slower and less vigorous; the secondary response, due to memory, is characterized by a more rapid and vigorous response (Figure 1.1). This is also the rationale behind vaccination – a relatively harmless form of pathogen (e.g. a killed virus) is used to invoke a primary response and imprint memory: any subsequent contact with the pathogen results in a secondary response, which is early and more vigorous.

Specificity implies that contact with one pathogen does not confer protection against other pathogens: the immune system differentiates specifically between two organisms. *Diversity* is an essential component of the adaptive immune system since the environment is full of millions of potential pathogens, yet the immune system demonstrates a remarkable capacity to mount a response to most of them. This diversity of the immune system is an essential feature if the body is to combat infection successfully. The basis of this diversity is dealt with later in the section on the genetics of the immune response. *Tolerance* to 'self' is an essential component of the immune system, since the system must not only distinguish between two pathogens, but must also distinguish between 'self' and 'non-self'. Occasionally the system breaks down and autoimmunity develops, and this issue is explored further in Chapter 5. The tolerance to self-antigens is established in early life, before maturation of the immune system: those circulating body components which reach the developing lymphoid system in the perinatal period induce a permanent self-tolerance, so that when immune maturity is established, there is an inability to respond to self-components.

INNATE AND ADAPTIVE IMMUNE SYSTEMS: AN INTIMATE INTERACTION

The division between the innate and acquired immune systems is largely for clarity and convenience. In practice, there is such an intimate interaction between the two systems that it is misleading to consider them as two separate entities. Therefore, in the rest of this chapter, the distinction between the two is largely abandoned and the essential components of the immune system are described in terms of functional phenotype. Thus, the description is based on the following:

(1) *Cells involved in the immune system:* this includes the professional phagocytes and natural killer (NK) cells considered to be part of the innate system, as well as the T cells and B cells, usually considered part of the adaptive system;

(2) *Molecules/humoral components of the immune system:* this includes antibodies, the T cell receptor, major histocompatibility complex (MHC) antigens, complement, acute-phase proteins and cytokines;

(3) *Effector functions in the immune system* are then described showing how the various components of the immune system interact with each other to mount an immune response.

CELLS INVOLVED IN IMMUNE REACTIONS

Lymphocytes and *phagocytes*, which originate from bone-marrow stem cells (Figure 1.2), are the predominant cells of the immune system, and they interact with each

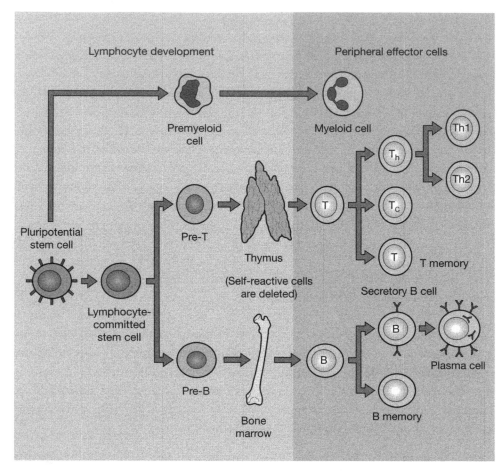

Figure 1.2 Development of different types of lymphocytes from a pluripotential stem cell in the bone marrow

other and other cells of the body to generate the immune response. Various leukocyte populations can be identified via their morphology and the molecules expressed on the cell surface, which are recognizable with monoclonal antibodies. Such molecules are termed *markers*, and a system of nomenclature has been devised for all the major molecules. This is called the cluster of differentiation (CD) system. While CD molecules allow the identification of leukocyte subpopulations, it has become clear that they subserve specific functions, e.g. the molecule CD3, found on all mature T cells, is associated with the antigen receptor and acts in transducing activation signals to the cell. Some CD molecules may appear transiently during lymphocyte development (e.g. the CD1 molecule on cortical thymocytes), or following cellular activation (e.g. the interleukin-2 receptor CD25), while others are stable and

Table 1.1 Key markers of lymphocyte populations

Marker function	Immuno-globulin antigen receptor	TcR/CD3 T cell activator	CD4 MHC class II binding	CD8 MHC class II binding	CD8 MHC class I binding	CD5
B cells	+	−	−	−	−	+/−*
T_h cells†	−	+	+	+	−	+
T_C cells†	−	+	+	−	+	+

T_h, helper T cells; T_C, cytotoxic T cells; TcR, T cell receptor; MHC, major histocompatibility complex
* a minor subpopulation of B cells is CD+
† the great majority of helper T cells are CD4+ and the majority of suppressors and cytotoxics, CD8+; exceptions have been found

expressed on particular cell lineages. The key markers of leukocyte subpopulations are listed in Table 1.1.

Professional phagocytes

Mononuclear phagocytes are widely distributed throughout the body. They are diverse, including not only blood monocytes, but also microglia of the brain and the Kupffer cells of the liver. Blood monocytes can migrate into the tissues where they develop into macrophages. The latter express receptors for immunoglobulin and complement components, and may be activated by cytokines released from T cells. Their surface molecules facilitate binding to antigens and subsequent phagocytosis. Internalized material (e.g. viruses) is broken down within phagolysosomes (cytoplasmic vesicles) and converted into peptides, which can be recycled to the surface to be presented to T cells by MHC molecules. Macrophages are relatively long-lived. Some return from the periphery to secondary lymphoid tissues, thereby transporting antigen from the periphery into the spleen and lymph nodes. An essential function of these cells is the internal destruction of pathogens and antigens.

Natural killer cells

These cells are considered part of the innate immune system, and although grouped as one, in fact there are different kinds of NK cells with somewhat different properties. In recent years, NK cells have attracted a great deal of attention from reproductive immunobiologists, as a particular form of NK cell constitutes the predominant

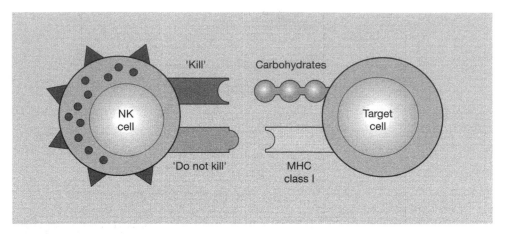

Figure 1.3 Recognition of the target cell by natural killer (NK) cells. The current thinking is that killing by NK cells requires two signals: a 'kill' signal and the absence of a 'do not kill' signal. The 'do not kill' signal seems to be the expression of major histocompatibility complex (MHC) class I molecules on the surface of the potential target, because cells that express MHC I cannot usually be killed by NK cells. The 'kill' signal is thought to involve interactions between proteins on the surface of NK cells and special carbohydrates on the surface of the target cell

population in the uterine decidua, and may well play an important role in pregnancy outcome. It is well established that with regard to peripheral NK cells, both the number and killing capacity decrease during normal pregnancy, and it has been suggested that high numbers and/or activity may predispose to implantation failure and/or recurrent miscarriage (see Chapter 3).

Within tissues, NK cells demonstrate significant versatility in their actions. They can kill tumor cells, virus-infected cells, bacteria, fungi and parasites. They kill by at least two methods. They can bore a hole in a target cell by secreting perforin molecules to form a membrane attack complex (see also under 'Complement' on p. 10) on the surface of the target. The NK cell can then secrete enzymes that enter the target cell and cause it to commit suicide. The second method of killing employs a protein called Fas ligand (FasL) that is expressed on the NK cell surface. FasL can interact with a protein called Fas on the surface of the target cell, and when the two proteins interact, they can signal the target cell to commit suicide by apoptosis.

NK cells do not have the equivalent of the T cell receptor (see below), and the mechanism by which they recognize their target has yet to be fully elucidated. However, the most popular theory suggests that two signals are involved, the so-called 'kill' signal, and the absence of the 'do not kill' signal. The 'kill' signal is thought to involve interactions between proteins on the surface of the NK cell and special carbohydrates on the surface of the target, which may indicate infection with a virus, or that a cell has become malignant. The 'do not kill' signal seems to be the expression of MHC class I molecules on the surface of potential target cells, since cells that express MHC class I usually cannot be killed by NK cells. The balance between the two signals determines whether NK cells will kill a target cell (Figure 1.3).

It is clearly advantageous to have cells that can kill targets which do not express MHC class I molecules, since many viruses and malignant cells can turn off the expression of MHC: these infected or malignant cells would therefore evade destruction by killer T cells (see below), and the NK cells would act as an all-important back-up system to avoid such a scenario. Additional fascinating features of NK cells include the fact that, unlike T cells which need 'thymic education' to avoid attacking self (see below), NK cells do not appear to need this education. NK cells also have properties of both cytotoxic T lymphocytes (CTLs) and helper T cells, since they not only use perforin and FasL to kill, just like CTLs, but they also produce large amounts of cytokines (especially interferon-γ (IFN-γ)), just like helper T cells. In other ways, NK cells resemble macrophages: they contain large amounts of lysosome-like granules, and can exist in several stages of readiness. Resting NK cells are able to produce some IFN-γ, but they produce more IFN-γ and kill more efficiently when activated. NK cells can be activated by lipopolysaccharide (LPS), which can also activate macrophages. They can also be activated by the signals IFN-α and IFN-β, which are released by cells under viral attack.

B lymphocytes

B lymphocytes are characterized by their expression of surface immunoglobulin (antibody), which acts as a receptor for antigen. They recognize native antigens in solution or on the surface of other cells. B cells, activated by contact with their specific antigen and triggered by cytokines released from T cells, divide and differentiate into antibody-secreting plasma cells. The secreted antibody is of identical antigen specificity to that on the original B cell, although it may become refined during the development of an immune response, resulting in an increasing affinity for the antigen. Antibodies are classified into different biochemical classes (see below). Virgin B cells initially express immunoglobulin M (IgM) with or without IgD on their surface. During B cell differentiation, individual cells may switch to the production of IgG, IgA or IgE, while retaining the antigen specificity.

T lymphocytes

T lymphocytes mature in the thymus, and three major events occur during thymic differentiation:

Table 1.2   Characteristics of antigen-presenting cells

Cell type	Location	MHC class II	Antigen presentation
Langerhans cell	skin	+	weak
Veiled cell	afferent lymph	+	
Interdigitating dendritic cell	lymph node, T cell areas	+	strong immunostimulation of resting T cells
Non-lymphoid dendritic cell	connective tissues of most organs	+	? T cells
Follicular dendritic cell	lymph node follicles	–	B cells
Mononuclear phagocytes and macrophages	many tissues	$0 \rightarrow ++$	B cells and primed T cells
Marginal zone macrophages	marginal zone of spleen and lymph nodes	–/+	T-independent antigens to B cells
B cells	lymphoid tissue	$+ \rightarrow ++$	to primed T cells

MHC, major histocompatibility complex

(1)   The development of a repertoire of T cell receptors (TcRs), and preferential selection of cells carrying TcRs that may interact effectively with the individual's MHC molecules in antigen presentation;

(2)   The selective removal of cells that recognize the individual's own molecules (i.e. self-antigens);

(3)   The differentiation of various T cell subpopulations.

T cell precursors entering the thymus lack specific T cell markers. They acquire CD2 at an early stage of development, and this is retained in mature T cells. Immature thymocytes express both CD4 and CD8, but one of these markers is lost as the cells mature. Thus, T cells leaving the thymus express either CD4 or CD8. A considerable selective pressure is exerted at this stage, and the large majority of thymocytes die without completing differentiation into mature T cells. T cell subpopulations have been identified by functional studies or using markers. At least two major sets are described: helper T cells (T_h), predominantly CD4+; and cytotoxic T cells (T_C), mostly CD8+. T cells recognize antigens (as peptide fragments) on the surface of other cells, in association with molecules encoded by the MHC (see below). The process by which cells express molecules recognizable by T cells is termed antigen presentation, and the cells are antigen-presenting cells (APCs). Many cell types are

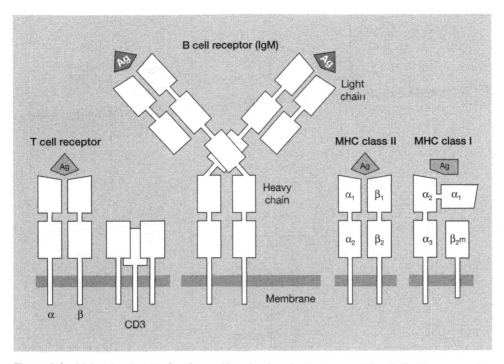

Figure 1.4 Molecules that bind antigens. Note the domain structure and the similarities among the molecules belonging to the immunoglobulin supergene family. Ag, antigen; IgM, Immunoglobulin M; MHC, major histocompatibility complex

capable of presenting antigens in a recognizable form to both B and T lymphocytes, and are thus collectively described as APCs (Table 1.2). CD8+ T cells recognize antigen in association with MHC class I molecules, and CD4+ cells recognize antigen in association with MHC class II molecules. T cell activation causes the cells to divide and secrete various cytokines that modulate immune responses. In addition, cytotoxic T cells secrete molecules called perforins, which polymerize to form holes in the membranes of target cells.

MOLECULES/HUMORAL ELEMENTS INVOLVED IN IMMUNE REACTIONS

Complement, acute-phase proteins and lysozyme are part of the innate immune system, and are key players in the immune response. Three groups of molecules are intimately involved in antigen-binding, namely antibodies, TcRs and MHC molecules (Figure 1.4). Antibodies recognize antigen alone, while TcRs recognize antigen plus

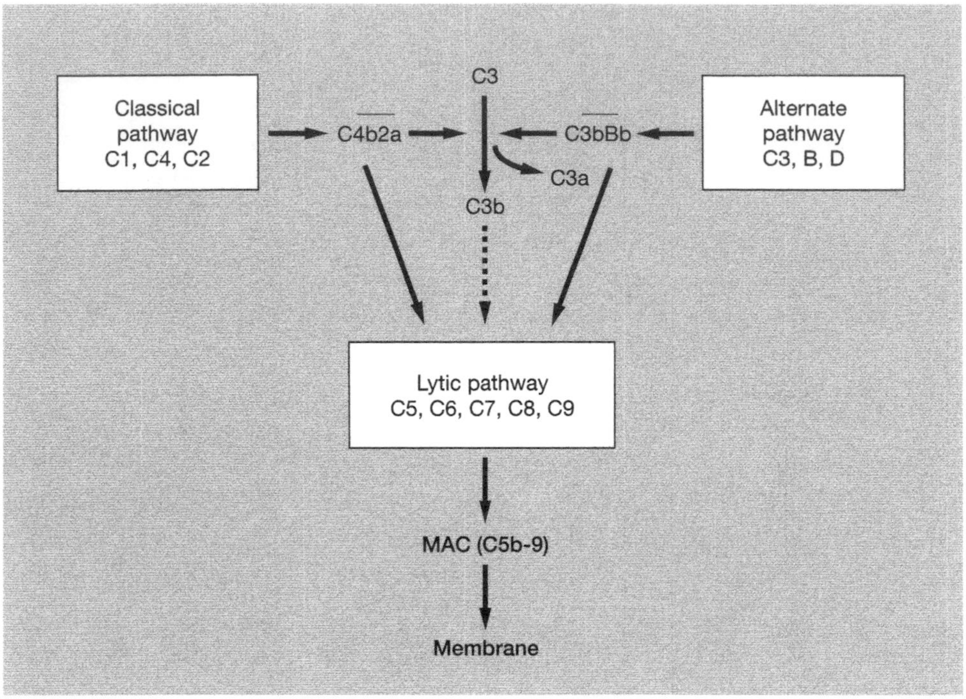

Figure 1.5 Complement pathways. Complement pathways may be activated by antigen–antibody complexes via the classic pathway or via the alternative pathway. Both routes generate a C3 convertase, which splits C3 into C3a and C3b. C3b deposited on an activator surface in association with a C3 convertase can initiate the lytic pathway to deposit membrane attack complexes (MACs) onto the target membrane

MHC, and both are highly specific in their binding. MHC molecules bind peptides which they present to T cells.

Cytokines are central to the regulation of the immune response, and although classically secreted by T cells, in fact a wide range of cells, including non-immune cells of the uterine epithelium, can and do secrete. This illustrates the futility of dividing the immune system into an innate and an adaptive component.

Complement

Complement is a system of more than 30 interacting proteins and their receptors. There are two pathways by which complement can be activated: the classical pathway involves antibody–antigen complexes, and the alternative pathway involves the presence of activator surfaces. Activators in the alternative pathway include certain microbial cell walls, carbohydrates and viruses. Complement activation is a complex process, but can be conveniently summarized as depicted in Figure 1.5. Activation can lead to the covalent attachment of a fragment of the third component of the system (i.e. C3b) to the initiating agent. Mononuclear phagocytes and neutrophils express receptors (mainly CR1 and CR3) for this fragment; thus, complement deposition on particles or antigen–antibody complexes opsonizes them for phagocytosis. The binding of C3b to receptors on phagocytes increases their level of activation, thereby priming them to eliminate the material they have phagocytosed.

The deposition of C3b on membranes can lead to activation of the complement lytic pathway. This involves the assembly of a membrane attack complex (MAC) that contains components which range from C5 through to C9 and traverse the membranes of the target cell. If MACs become assembled on eukaryotic cells (e.g. on an erythrocyte), they cause osmotic damage to the cells and can lead to their lysis. Other complement components are involved in development of the inflammatory reaction, when they act as anaphylatoxins, inducing smooth muscle contraction and mast cell degranulation, and being chemotactic for neutrophils and macrophages. This is thought to be important in control of the initial influx of phagocytes into sites of acute inflammation.

Cytokines

Cytokines are soluble proteins released by one cell that act on receptors on other cells to affect their functions. Thus, many of the interactions between cells co-operating or participating in an immune response are controlled by cytokines. Cytokine activity is not confined to classical immune responses, and as more and more cytokines are discovered, it becomes increasingly apparent that their actions are wide, complex and intertwined with a wide range of other biological interactions within an organism. Several cytokines may have the same effect, or they may act synergistically, the action of one potentiating the actions of another; for example IFN-γ induces MHC class II on many cells, and this effect is enhanced by tumor necrosis factor-α (TNFα), while TNFα itself has no class II-inducing ability; interleukin-1 (IL-1), released by macrophages and a number of other cells, enhances the level of IL-2 receptors on the T cell, while IL-2 maintains T cells in the cell cycle. Table 1.3 lists the known functions of the more important cytokines.

Immunoglobulins

Antibodies (or immunoglobulins) have a basic structure consisting of four polypeptide chains (Figure 1.6). There are two identical heavy chains and two identical light chains that are linked by disulfide bonds and non-covalent interactions. Each of

Table 1.3 Major cytokines and their functions

Cytokine	Sources	Targets	Principal effects
IL-1	macrophages, LGLs, B cells	lymphocytes macrophages endothelium tissue cells	activation and IL-2 receptor induction activation increased leukocyte adhesion numerous effects in inflammatory reactions
IL-2	T cells	T cells active B cells	T cell division and differentiation; absolute requirement promotes B cell division
IL-4 and IL-5	T cells	B cells	required for B cell division and differentiation
IL-6	T cells lymphocytes macrophages fibroblasts	B cells hepatocytes	B cell differentiation acute-phase protein synthesis
IFN-γ	T cells	leukocytes endothelium tissue cells	macrophage activation increased leukocyte adhesion MHC induction
TNFα	macrophages	phagocytes	activation
TNFβ	T cells	K and NK cells endothelium target cells	activation promotes leukocyte adhesion increased susceptibility to cytotoxic cells
IL-3	T cells	stem cells	control stem cell division and differentiation pathways
M-CSF	mononuclear cells	stem cells	control stem cell division and differentiation pathways
G-CSF	endothelium		
GM-CSF	T cells mononuclear cells endothelium fibroblasts	stem cells	control stem cell division and differentiation pathways

IL, interleukin; LGLs, large granular lymphocytes; IFN, interferon; TNF, tumor necrosis factor; CSF, colony-stimulating factor; M, macrophage; G, granulocyte; GM, granulocyte-macrophage; K, killer; NK, natural killer; MHC, major histocompatibility complex

these chains is formed by a number of globular domains connected by less tightly folded regions of polypeptide chains.

Light chains have two domains and heavy chains four or five, depending on the class of antibody. Each four-polypeptide unit has two antigen-combining sites, formed by the N-terminal domains, causing them to be very variable between antibodies, the greatest variability being clustered at the extreme ends of the domains where antigen binds. These domains are thus called variable or V domains, while the

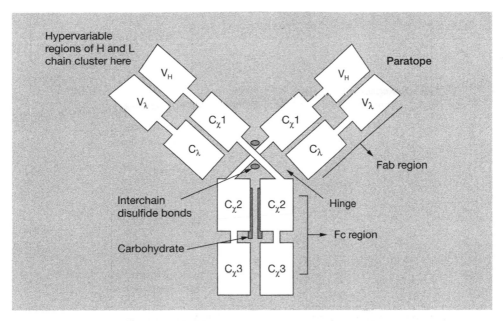

Figure 1.6 Structure of immunoglobulin (Ig). The structual details of an IgG molecule are illustrated with the names of the domains and different areas of the molecule noted. Interchain disulfide bonds are marked. In this example the light chains are λ

segments of polypeptide that show the greatest variability (three per V domain) are called hypervariable regions. These hypervariable regions are not contiguous in the polypeptide chain, but are brought into proximity at the antigen-binding site by the overall folding of the polypeptide chain within the domain. The antigen-binding site is sometimes called the antibody paratope, in accordance with the naming of an antigenic determinant as an epitope. With six different hypervariable regions of different amino acid sequence at the paratope (three from the heavy chain, three from the light), the molecular surfaces of different antibodies are highly variable in shape, charge and amino acid residues; this gives them their antigen specificity.

The remaining domains are less variable between antibodies and are called constant or C domains, but even here there is some variability. Light chains may be one of two different types, namely kappa (κ) or lambda (λ), that are generated from two different gene loci. The heavy chain gene locus in the human can generate nine different types of heavy chains that vary in their three domains (in addition to the huge amounts of variation seen in the V domains), and there is a gene for each of these chains. This allows for the formation of antibody isotypes, termed μ, δ, γ1, γ2, γ3, γ4, α1, α2 and ε. The heavy chain isotype present in an antibody determines the class and subclass of that antibody. Any one of these isotypes can be produced in a membrane-bound form to act as a B cell antigen receptor, or in a secreted form to

Table 1.4 Antibody characteristics and functions

Class	H2L2 sub-units	H-chain domains	Iso-types	C1q binding	Placental transfer	Cellular binding	Serum concentration in adult (mg/ml)
IgG	1	4	IgG1	++	+	neutrophils, MOs	9
			IgG2	+	(+)	neutrophils, MOs weak	3
			IgG3	+++	+	neutrophils, MOs	1
			IgG4	–	+	neutrophils, MOs weak	0.5
IgA	1 or 2	4	IgA1	–	–	neutrophils	3
						neutrophils	0.5
IgM	5	5	IgM	+++	–		1.5
IgD	1	4	IgD	–	–		0.03
IgE	1	5	IgE	–	–	mast cells, basophils, MOs weak	0.00005

Ig, immunoglobulin; MOs, mononuclear cells; H2L2, heavy and light chains

become part of the effector arm of the immune response. Antibodies can be divided into five classes, or nine subclasses, corresponding to the nine isotypes (Table 1.4). The immunoglobulin G (IgG) class has four isotypes (IgG1, IgG2, IgG3 and IgG4) and the IgA class two subclasses (IgA1 and IgA2), and IgD, IgM and IgE classes are not usually subdivided. While all antibodies can bind antigen, each antibody class, and indeed subclass, has a different set of functions. These functions relate to the capacity of the constant regions of the antibody to interact with different tissues expressing Fc (crystallizable fragment of immunoglobulin) receptors, or with C1q of the complement system. Antibodies are therefore bifunctional molecules in which the V domains are responsible for antigen binding, while the C domains allow inter-action with various effector systems.

The T cell receptor

The TcR is an integral membrane protein consisting of a pair of polypeptide chains linked by a disulfide bond. Four genetic loci (α, β, γ, δ) encode these polypeptide chains, and a T cell may have either an $\alpha\beta$ pair (TcR2) or a $\gamma\delta$ pair (TcR1). Most mature peripheral T cells have TcR2, while TcR1 receptors are seen on a population of thymic T cells and on some T cells located in the peripheral lymphoid tissues, such as those in the gut. The functional significance of there being two different

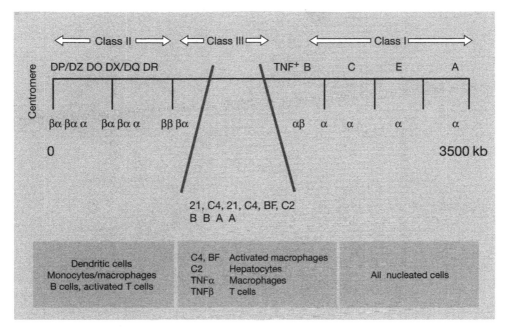

Figure 1.7 Major histocompatibility complex. Class I genes encoded the α/β heterodimer. The β chain (β₂-microglobulin) is on a different chromosome. The α and β chain genes for class II occur in pairs. Class III genes encode four components of the complement system but genes encoding 21-hydroxylase A and B are located in the same region. Tumor necrosis factor (TNF+), α and β genes; BF, factor B

types of TcRs is not known. The polypeptide chains each have two extracellular domains, of which the N-terminal domains are variable (V) and form the MHC antigen recognition site. Each TcR is associated with a number of other polypeptide chains in the cell membrane, and these associated polypeptides (denoted γ, δ, ε) appear to be involved in transducing the activation signal to the cell via calcium, and are referred to as the CD3 complex. The CD3 chains are monomorphic and distinct from the chains that form the TcR.

The major histocompatibility complex

The MHC is the human leukocyte antigen (HLA) locus on chromosome 6, and its products are termed MHC antigens or molecules (synonymous with HLA). The MHC can be divided into three distinct regions encoding three classes of molecules (Figure 1.7). The A, B and C loci (class I genes) encode class I molecules; the DP, DQ and DR loci (class II genes) encode class II molecules; and the class III genes encode a variety of other molecules with diverse functions. The class I loci each encode the α chain of a single class I molecule. Class II molecules have two

15

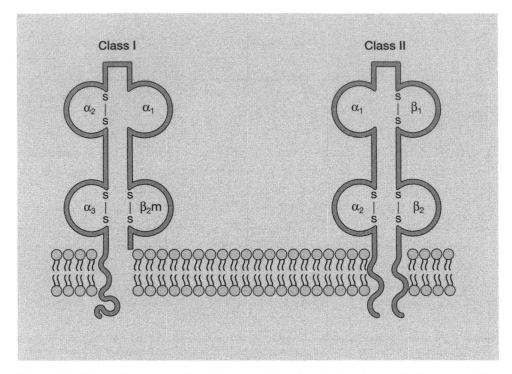

Figure 1.8 Schematic representation of class I and class II molecules of the major histocompatibility complex MHC. Note the globular domain structure

polypeptide chains, and there are one or more genes for each pair of chains in each class II locus.

The MHC class I and class II molecules share a common molecular ancestry with the domains of immunoglobulin and TcR, and are thus members of the immunoglobulin supergene family of molecules. They are cell-surface glycoproteins, each of which has four external domains (Figure 1.8). Class I molecules have one polypeptide chain (α) encoded within the MHC. Each chain folds into three extracellular domains which are linked non-covalently to the molecule β_2-microglobulin, the latter making the fourth domain of the class I molecule. MHC class II molecules each consist of two polypeptides (α and β), both encoded in the MHC. They are non-covalently associated and both traverse the membrane. MHC molecules are highly polymorphic (i.e. there is a great deal of genetic variation between individuals). For example, there are at least 50 structural variants of the HLA-B molecule, and at least 25 HLA-DR variants. Each of these variants may occur with any combination of the others, thus allowing for a vast number of potential different MHC haplotypes.

MHC molecules are involved in presenting antigen to T cells. Different MHC molecules present different antigens more effectively than others. Consequently, it is advantageous to carry a wide range of MHC molecules that can present the numerous antigens that may be encountered. Analysis of the polypeptide structure of MHC molecules shows that the variability is concentrated in regions in the two domains that are furthest from the membrane, that is the α_1 and β_2 domains of class I molecules and the N-terminal domains of the α and β chains of the class II molecules.

Following crystallographic analysis of class I molecules, the structure of MHC molecules has recently begun to be elucidated. HLA-A2 molecules have the two domains nearest the membranes folded in a broadly similar way to the immunoglobulin domains, but the more variable distal domains form a peptide-binding site, consisting of a base of β-pleated sheet surrounded and enclosed by two loops of an α-helix, one on each side of the binding sites. These loops contain the regions of greatest sequence variability between different class I variants. It is thought that the residues facing into the binding site will determine how the molecule binds to peptides, while residues pointing outwards will control interactions of the MHC antigen complex with the TcR. There is a considerable amount of structural similarity between the class I and II molecules, particularly with respect to the regions surrounding the binding site, and there is increasing evidence to suggest functional similarity between the two classes of molecule.

EFFECTOR FUNCTIONS IN THE IMMUNE RESPONSE

The theory of clonal selection

The fundamental challenge for the immune system is to be able to protect the body against an almost infinite range of pathogens, some of which have the capacity to mutate to evade immune recognition and therefore immune responses. It is now generally accepted that this capacity is based on clonal activation. The basis of an immune response is the stimulation and activation of clones of lymphocytes capable of recognizing the initiating antigen. Although there is only a modest number of genes for immunoglobulin and TcRs, a complex process of genetic recombination generates an enormous diversity of receptors (see 'Suggested further reading', p. 20). Since this occurs during lymphocyte ontogeny, antigen is not required to generate the repertoire of receptors. Each lymphocyte expresses a receptor of only one specificity, and the entire repertoire is only present when one considers the total population of lymphocytes within the body. It is therefore evident that the system generates receptors for a vast number of antigens, of which the great majority may never be encountered in a lifetime. One consequence of this diversity is that the proportion of lymphocytes expressing receptors for a particular antigen is relatively small. Thus, to mount an effective immune response, one of the first steps is the expansion

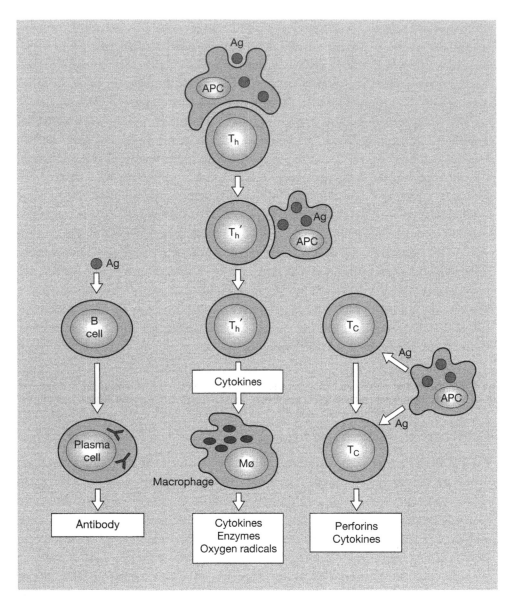

Figure 1.9 Overview of the immune response. Antigen (Ag) taken up by the antigen-presenting cells (APC) stimulates helper T cells (T_h) so that when they encounter the antigen again, they proliferate and release cytokines. These are involved in the differentation of B cells into antibody-producing plasma cells, the activation of macrophages (Mø), and the proliferation and activation of cytotoxic T cells (T_C), which recognize antigen on antigen-presenting target cells and can kill them by the action of perforins and cytokines

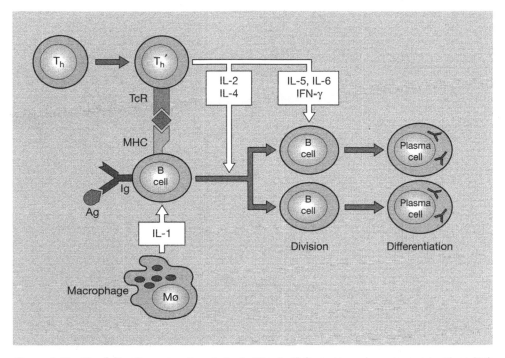

Figure 1.10   T cell–B cell co-operation. Activated T cells (T$_h$′) can recognize processed antigen (Ag) on B cells associated with major histocompatibility complex (MHC) class II molecules. Interleukin-2 (IL-2) released by macrophages (Mø), in associaton with IL-4 and IL-2 from the T cells, promotes B cell division and additional cytokines then promote differentiation into plasma cells. Ig, immunoglobulin; TcR, T cell receptor; IFN, interferon

of clones of antigen-reactive cells. In effect, antigen selects and activates those lymphocytes that recognize it. This is called the theory of clonal selection.

Cellular interactions in immune reactions

Figure 1.9 depicts an overview of events occurring during an immune response. The interactions of B cells and macrophages with T cells are particularly important in development of the immune response. The critical events include: antigen uptake and processing by antigen-presenting cells; antigen presentation to and recognition by antigen-specific B and/or T cells; co-operation between T and B cells (Figure 1.10), with release of cytokines that subserve a variety of functions including induction of B-cell differentiation and macrophage activation; and the development of cytotoxic activity (Figure 1.11). Antibodies produced by plasma cells may neutralize pathogens by direct binding (e.g. blocking viral receptors), but more often they link antigen to cells of the immune system, or activate the complement system. Many of

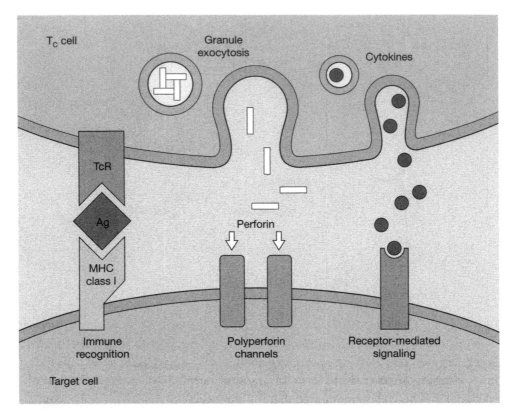

Figure 1.11 Actions of cytotoxic T cells (T$_C$). T$_C$ cells recognize targets primarily by major histocompatibility complex (MHC) class I-mediated interactions. They can then damage the target cell by release of perforins, which polymerize to form polyperforin channels, or via other molecules released by the cytotoxic cell, including some cytokines. TcR, T cell receptor; Ag, antigen

the effects of antibody occur via binding to Fc receptors, which bind to sites in the constant domains of the antibody.

SUGGESTED FURTHER READING

Playfair JHL, Chain BM, Immunology at a Glance, 7th edition. Oxford: Blackwell Science, 2003

Roitt IM. Essential Immunology, 9th edition. Oxford: Blackwell Science, 1992

Sompayrac LM. How the Immune System Works. Oxford: Blackwell Science, 1999

2

The immunological paradox of pregnancy

2.1 Maternal immunology

A BRIEF HISTORY

In the preceding chapter on the essentials of basic immunology, it is clear that a fundamental requirement of the immune system is that it can distinguish normal healthy cells (*self*) from *non-self* (infected, malignant or allogeneic cells and toxins). Some 50 years ago, working on the biology of transplantation, Peter Medawar and his colleagues discovered the laws of transplantation immunology. Put simply, Medawar and his colleagues showed that it is impossible to transplant grafts between genetically dissimilar individuals (Figure 2.1). They further demonstrated that graft rejection is an immunological phenomenon – they demonstrated specificity, memory and primary and secondary kinetics in graft rejection responses. Further research was later to demonstrate that antigens of the major histocompatibility complex (MHC) elicited the strongest rejection responses (hence human leukocyte antigens (HLAs) were initially termed *transplantation antigens*).

It should not perhaps be surprising that for a philosopher–scientist of Medawar's stature, the survival of the mammalian fetus – whose allograft status is conferred by the inheritance of histocompatibility and red blood cell antigens from the father – posed an obvious and compelling challenge to the laws of transplantation immunology. It is well known now that the more outbred a population, the more vigorous the offspring, and studies from 'closed' communities show that consanguineous marriages preserve deleterious recessive genes and result in less robust offspring. Medawar first drew attention to this apparent challenge in a lecture he delivered to the Society of Experimental Biology, and he subsequently wrote this in what has become a landmark paper entitled: 'Some immunological and endocrinological problems raised by the evolution of viviparity in vertebrates'. Medawar paraphrased the conundrum thus:

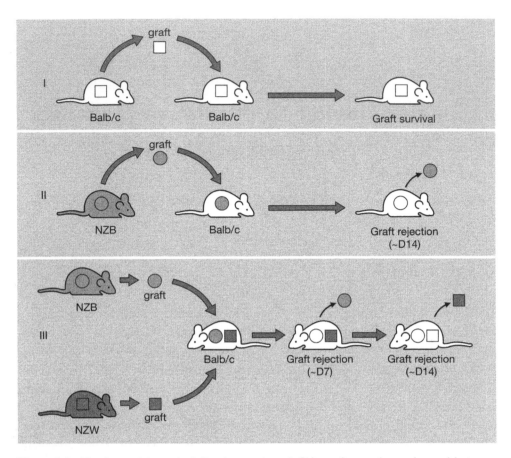

Figure 2.1 The laws of transplantation immunology. I. Skin grafts can be exchanged between genetically similar mice (Balb/c to Balb/c). II. When a skin graft from a NZB mouse is transplanted onto a Balb/c mouse, the graft is rejected at about 2 weeks. III. When the same recipient Balb/c mouse is transplanted with two types of graft, one from the same NZB mouse as in II above, and another from a NZW mouse, both grafts are rejected, but due to the previous priming/sensitization, the graft from the NZB mouse is rejected at a much earlier stage. Graft rejection is an immunological phenomenon, showing primary and secondary responses. Antibodies to donor antigens can be demonstrated in the recipient following rejection, and immune cells can be found in the rejection graft. The basis of the graft rejection is the disparity in the major histocompatibility complex (MHC) antigens between the donor and recipient – hence MHC antigens were once referred to as 'transplantation antigens'. On the face of it, human pregnancy would appear to defy all the basic laws of transplantation immunology: the more outbred a population, the more vigorous the offspring; second and subsequent babies tend on average to be bigger than the first; but while there is no good evidence of a cellular immunological reaction against the fetus, anti-MHC antibodies are frequently demonstrated in the sera of multiparous women

'...how does the pregnant mother contrive to nourish within itself, for many weeks or months, the foetus that is an antigenically foreign body? Is pregnancy accompanied by any physiological changes which may in some degree prevent the foetus, qua tissue homograph, from immunising the mother against itself?'

This intriguing situation gave rise to concepts such as the 'immunological paradox' of pregnancy, the fetus being regarded as 'nature's perfect allograft'. Many scientists thought that the unraveling of nature's secrets would result in great strides being made in various fields, including transplantation and tumor immunology, not to mention human reproduction and advances in basic science. Medawar himself, always the philosopher–scientist, offered three possible hypotheses:

(1) That there may be an anatomical separation of the fetus from the mother;

(2) That the fetus may be antigenically immature;

(3) That the mother may be immunologically indolent.

Although in his theoretical treatise, Medawar explored these possibilities with his characteristic clarity and incisiveness, alas he was never to conduct a single laboratory experiment to address this specific issue. He was to produce further sterling work with colleagues such as Leslie Brent and Rupert Billingham on the cellular basis of transplantation and the induction of specific tolerance, for which he was jointly awarded the Nobel Prize for Medicine in 1960 with another giant of immunology, Macfarlane Burnet. But Medawar's seminal publication had heralded the birth of 'reproductive immunology', and as seen below, his own conclusion that the single most important factor ensuring the survival of the fetal semiallograft is the anatomical separation of the fetus from its mother remains the most cogent and convincing explanation. He is thus often referred to as the father of reproductive immunology. What should be made of his speculations on the possible mechanisms of survival of the fetus? It is as well to discard those hypotheses that have been categorically shown to be unsustainable. It is now clear that the fetus is antigenically mature from an early stage, and that immunocompetence begins to develop in the first trimester of pregnancy. Although there is some modulation of the maternal immune response during pregnancy, in fact the mother remains immunocompetent, certainly so that she could not possibly ignore as powerful a potential immunogen as an allograft. The issue of the anatomical separation of fetus from mother, and possible maternal immunological indolence, is explored in greater detail below.

In the late 1950s and early 1960s, the concept of 'immunological privilege' – that certain parts of the body (such as the anterior chamber of the eye, the brain and the hamster cheek pouch) are not accessed by or lack elements of the immune response, and are therefore immunologically privileged – was well established. Billingham, Medawar's erstwhile colleague, suggested that perhaps the uterus too was immunologically privileged, thus giving a fourth possible explanation for the survival of the fetus. However, attractive as it was as a hypothesis, it is now well established that the uterus is not immunologically privileged: it has an extensive lymphatic and vascular network, especially prominent during pregnancy. Furthermore, elegant experiments using mammalian systems have shown that allografts placed in the uterus are rejected in much the same way as when placed in other sites, and that pre-existing systemic allograft immunity can be expressed within the decidua.

Although the concept of the 'fetal allograft' has dominated ideas and thinking in reproductive immunology, not only is it clear that the fetus should not be regarded as a conventional allograft, but more recent research has demonstrated an important role for the innate system in the maternofetal immunological relationship, and it is likely that this relationship will need redefinition.

FRONTIERS OF IMMUNOLOGICAL CONFRONTATION IN HUMAN REPRODUCTION

It is important to recognize that it is not just the survival of the fetus that needs explanation in immunological terms, but there are other areas of potential immunological confrontation that must be addressed in trying to understand the apparent immunological paradox of pregnancy, and they include the following:

(1) Immunity to sperm and seminal fluid;

(2) How the preimplantation embryo evades the maternal immune system;

(3) Implantation and placentation: the nature of the maternofetal immunological interface;

(4) Maternal immunocompetence during pregnancy;

(5) Maternal immune responses to fetal antigens;

(6) Whether recurrent miscarriage represents failure of ill-defined immunoregulatory mechanisms that normally sustain successful pregnancy.

Current ideas on these and other issues are reviewed below.

Sperm and seminal plasma

Antigenicity of spermatozoa

A multiplicity of antigens can be demonstrated on sperm by fluorescent labeling using antibody produced in mice or rabbits. They tend to localize to and be specific for particular areas of the spermatozoon. Some antigens may only be revealed after capacitation. Whether MHC antigens are or are not expressed on sperm is still not definitively determined. The significance in human reproduction of sperm antigens is not entirely clear. Although some infertile men and women can be shown to possess antibodies against all of these regions, antibodies against surface antigens of the acrosome and main tailpiece seem to be of the greatest pathological relevance because they cause immobilization and/or agglutination of sperm.

Tolerance to self-sperm antigens

As discussed in Chapter 1, tolerance to self-antigens occurs as a result of suppression and/or elimination of potentially self-reactive T cells in the thymus during fetal life. Since spermatogenesis does not commence until long after this self-recognition process is over, spermatozoa should be particularly susceptible to the development of autoimmunity. This can arise and be a cause of male infertility, but in reality it is very rare indeed. Among the mechanisms which prevent antisperm autoimmunity from occurring more often are thought to be the following:

(1) Physical contact between immunocompetent cells and developing spermatozoa is prevented by the tight junctions between Sertoli cells lining the seminiferous tubules;

(2) These same tight junctions prevent the passage of circulating antibody into the tubules;

(3) Autoreactivity against the highly immunogenic epididymal sperm may be prevented by suppressor T cells in the epididymal epithelium;

(4) Once sperm leave the epididymis, they become coated with seminal plasma components including lactoferrin, which reduces their immunogenicity – which may be relevant both while the sperm are in the seminal vesicles and also once they are deposited in the female vagina.

Tolerance to sperm antigens in the female genital tract

Repeated coitus throughout reproductive life results in the female genital tract being frequently exposed to spermatozoa. The former possesses a mucosal immune system and can therefore mount immune responses, while spermatozoa are immunogenic, yet female genital tract antisperm immunity is a rare phenomenon! Clearly the prevention of an antisperm immune response is important for successful reproduction. There is now some evidence to suggest that seminal plasma has a powerful effect on most cells of the immune system and tends to impair the activity of both antibody and complement. Even low concentrations of seminal plasma *in vitro* can inhibit the generation of cytotoxic T cells, the cytotoxic effect of natural killer (NK) cells, the phagocytic activity of macrophages and neutrophils and the generation and activity

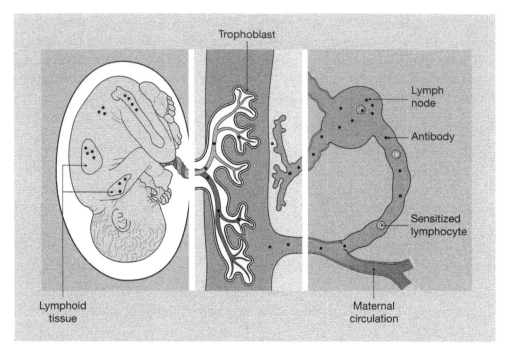

Figure 2.2 Anatomical relationship between mother and fetus

of antibodies. However, all this evidence has the disadvantage of being *in vitro*, and a biological significance for such effects cannot be assumed. Several of the immuno-suppressive components of seminal plasma have been characterized. Among these are zinc-containing compounds, the polyamines spermine and spermidine, prostaglandins, transglutaminases and a protein closely related to pregnancy-associated protein-A.

The preimplantation embryo

Following implantation, the zygote traverses the Fallopian tubes and enters the uterus. It represents the origins of the semiallograft, and is a potential immune target, and its survival needs explanation. It is now generally thought that protection of the preimplantation embryo depends primarily on the following:

(1) Paternal antigens are not expressed at the two-cell stage, but become apparent on the surface from the six-to-eight-cell stage;

(2) Although the expression of these antigens increases with cellular division, major histocompatibility antigens are thought not to be present at this stage in human pregnancy;

(3) Some research points to the existence of hormone-dependent non-specific suppressor cells in secretory-phase human endometrium. Supernatants from cultured explants of endometrium, which include these cells, have immunosuppressive effects. Thus, significant immunological problems are, therefore, not posed by the conceptus before implantation.

Immunology of implantation and placentation

The immunological enigma at the heart of viviparity becomes acute during and after implantation. The immunological relationship of mother and fetus is illustrated in Figure 2.2. In essence, the immunological problem exists because of the intimate juxtaposition of maternal and fetally derived tissue, which is at least partially foreign (semiallogeneic) to the mother. The following issues must now be considered to try to understand the nature of the maternofetal immunological relationship: the anatomy of the maternofetal interface; control of trophoblast growth; antigen expression by trophoblast; and immunology of the endometrium and decidua.

Anatomy of the maternofetal interface

A detailed description of the embryological development and the anatomical relationships of the interface is beyond the scope of this chapter; here are described those aspects that are relevant to immunological interactions. There is no vascular continuity between the fetal and maternal compartments. The fetus does not come into direct contact with maternal blood, but interacts via the placenta. The process of implantation and subsequent trophoblastic invasion culminates in an intimate interaction between trophoblast and decidua. Figure 2.2 depicts the possible interrelations between the various trophoblastic subpopulations. The syncytiotrophoblast, the non-mitotic outer layer of the chorionic villi, is bathed in maternal blood, as it also lines the intervillous spaces. Beneath the syncytiotrophoblast is the cytotrophoblast, whose cells are metabolically more active. Some cytotrophoblast cells push through the syncytiotrophoblast to make the cytotrophoblast columns which help anchor the villi to the maternal tissue, while other cytotrophoblast cells break away to form the cytotrophoblast shell, some of these cells subsequently migrating into the myometrium where they are called the interstitial cytotrophoblast cells. Other cytotrophoblast cells invade the spiral arterioles of the uterus and line the vessels as endovascular trophoblast. The cytotrophoblast and syncytiotrophoblast constitute the villous trophoblast. The non-villous trophoblast constitutes the rest of the trophoblast tissue, from which the chorion laeve and chorionic plate, the marginal zone and the basal plate of the placenta are formed. The trophoblast thus represents a continuous frontier over a considerable surface area, up to $15\,m^2$ at

20 weeks' gestation in human pregnancy. It has therefore long been the prime candidate for the role of an immunologically protective or insulating barrier.

Control of trophoblast growth

Very little is known currently about the mechanisms which control trophoblast growth and the development of its multiple functions. The next decade will undoubtedly see significant advances in the understanding of the fundamental processes involved in growth and differentiation in general. Knowledge of trophoblast growth and its control will also increase, not least because the human placenta is so readily available for study. There is experimental evidence to suggest that, in the mouse, decidual cells secrete substances which promote growth and development of trophoblast and other placental cells. Recent reports have provided at least a first glimpse of some very promising areas for future research. The first of these is in relation to proto-oncogenes, which are normal genes involved in cellular growth, proliferation and differentiation. Most of what is currently known about proto-oncogenes has been learnt from studying the rapidly transforming retroviruses. They carry specific genes (oncogenes) which are responsible for the viruses' oncogenic potential, and have been designated as, for example, *ras, myco, erb, fis* and *sis*. The puzzle arose when specific viral oncogenes (v-*onc*) were used as probes in normal tissue, including that of man, because the oncogenes were found to share some DNA amino acid sequences with those in normal cells. Why should this be so, since such a high degree of conservation of genetic material capable of inducing cancer would be such a disadvantage to the organism? Surely there must be some more fundamental and advantageous reason for the presence of these cellular oncogenes (c-*onc*)? This has led to the current thinking that, before viral conversion, the original genes (or proto-oncogenes) function in normal cellular proliferation or differentiation. Circumstantial evidence for this comes from the observation that, of the 20 known proto-oncogenes, at least three have been shown to be related to known growth factors or growth factor receptors. For example, the c-*sis* gene is associated with platelet derived growth factor, and the c-*erb* gene with epidermal growth factor receptor. The *myc* gene is also closely involved in cell proliferation. It is now thought that rapidly transforming retroviruses convert a normal growth gene into one which may be pathogenic, either by altering the gene structure to produce an abnormal gene product, or by amplification, thus increasing to abnormal levels the production of normal products.

The second exciting area is our burgeoning knowledge of the biological importance of growth factors (to which lymphokines and other cytokines belong) and their specific receptors on cells. Proto-oncogenes and growth factors seem to be functionally associated. Questions about their expression on trophoblast are obviously of great interest, and some answers are beginning to be produced. The proto-oncogenes c-*myc* and c-*sis* have been found to be co-expressed on extravillous cytotrophoblast. There is evidence that *myc* protein expression and epidermal growth factor (EGF) receptors are associated with trophoblast proliferation and differentiation. EGF receptors are known to be present in large numbers in the human placenta, and more detailed studies have localized their expression to the microvillous membrane of syncytiotrophoblast throughout human pregnancy, its basolateral membrane (but only at term) and villous cytotrophoblast cells in the first trimester. As these cells proliferate and migrate towards the maternal tissues, there is a dramatic increase in EGF receptor expression. This is in contradistinction to insulin receptor expression, which is only to be found on syncytiotrophoblast.

There may be links between tissue differentiation and EGF receptor expression and function on the following basis: syncytiotrophoblast is a non-proliferative and terminally differentiated tissue which expresses EGF receptor; it arises from villous cytotrophoblast which also expresses EGF receptor; as villous cytotrophoblast differentiation alters within the proliferating cell columns, so the expression of EGF receptor decreases; EGF can stimulate the release of human chorionic gonadotropin and human placental lactogen from syncytiotrophoblast in culture; and villous trophoblast produces most, if not all, of the placental proteins and hormones. Extravillous trophoblast is, in that sense, functionally inert. In the light of the association between proto-oncogenes and growth factors on the one hand, and retroviruses on the other, it is relevant to note that normal human placentas (like those of other primates) contain retroviral particles. In addition, antisera to human syncytiotrophoblast membranes can cross-react with simian retrovirus-producing cell lines. The significance of these observations remains unclear, but they clearly warrant further exploration.

Another observation which may well be of fundamental importance to the development of the fetus as well as the trophoblast is that development of the mouse embryo depends on distinctive contributions from both parental genomes. Specifically, embryonic development is controlled by the preferential expression of maternal or paternal genes in the embryo, whereas trophoblast development depends on the preferential expression of paternal rather than maternal genes. The mechanism for this is probably differential methylation of genes between embryo and trophoblast. The insertion of a methyl group into the amino acid sequence of a gene causes translation to stop at that point. This is consistent with the clinical observation in human trophoblastic tumors that complete hydatidiform moles are usually genetically androgenetic. The next few years are likely to afford further and clearer insights into the molecular and genetic basis of growth, differentiation and development.

Antigen expression by trophoblast

MHC antigen expression by trophoblast The biology and role of MHC antigens has already been discussed in Chapter 1. The current view is that trophoblast does not express classical MHC antigens, and that it does express a class I monomorphic molecule, HLA-G. Most, if not all, of the HLA molecules expressed on trophoblast are HLA-G. The regulation of HLA-G expression appears to occur at various levels. The HLA-G gene is transcribed in normal villous and extravillous trophoblast, but not in syncytiotrophoblast. Villous trophoblast can translate the transcribed message into expressed protein. HLA-G mRNA is expressed in first-trimester cytotrophoblast and in term chorionic membrane cytotrophoblast, but is seen in low amounts, if at all, in syncytiotrophoblast from both first- and third-trimester placenta. Unlike most other cell types, cytotrophoblast cannot be stimulated to up-regulate expression of HLA by cytokines such as IFN-γ virus infection.

HLA-G: evolutional vestige, or shield against natural killer cells? What is the function of this molecule? It would be all too easy to regard it as an evolutionary vestige, a useless molecule which was not subjected to the forces of evolutionary selection because it posed no threat to the continuity of the species. Yet it is odd that regulatory mechanisms seen to have evolved for its expression. Why, for instance, does it only occur predominantly on trophoblast, and why only in certain subsets of trophoblast? If it were simply redundant, it might be expressed on a wider range of tissues along with classical MHC antigens. It has been proposed that HLA-G may play a role in the resistance to lysis by NK cells. The hypothesis is that, while lack of classical MHC antigens confers resistance to lysis by allospecific T cells, total lack of MHC antigens would render trophoblast susceptible to lysis by NK cells, which are thought to lyse cells on the basis of recognition of altered self-antigens or absence of self (see Chapter 1). A monomorphic antigen, such as HLA-G, would be recognized as self. This hypothesis will best be explored with transgenic mice expressing predetermined levels of HLA-G. However, there are immediate problems with this hypothesis: how does syncytiotrophoblast, which is devoid of all MHC antigens, escape cytotoxic damage by NK cells? Moreover, not all extravillous trophoblast within decidua express HLA-G, and they should therefore be susceptible to lysis. Nevertheless, this is a potentially exciting area of enquiry, not least because many questions on the nature and role of HLA-G, including whether it can present antigen, may be answered. Already there is intensive research activity to try and answer these questions and more. HLA-transgenic mice, HLA-G-transfected cells and the use of protein-targeting techniques will not be the obvious tools in the unraveling of the role of HLA-G.

Non-MHC antigen expression by trophoblast   The trophoblast clearly expresses a wide range of antigens, but it is evident that only those antigenic systems that exhibit polymorphism would be of interest to the issue of fetal survival, since they would allow the possibility of allogeneic differences between mother and fetus. Such systems include the erythrocyte antigenic systems (i.e. ABO, P, Rh, K) and placental alkaline phosphatase.

Erythrocyte antigenic systems   Human trophoblast does not express the A and B blood group antigens, but rhesus D is expressed. The paradoxical observation is that this rhesus factor antigen does not appear to sensitize rhesus-negative women, any such sensitization occurring only when placental disruption occurs, such as at parturition. The function of rhesus D on trophoblast is not known, nor the reason for its failure to sensitize. It has been surmised that lack of MHC class II at the maternofetal interface results in failure to present antigen (rhesus D) to helper T cells, and thus failure of antibody production. Perhaps the bottom line where erythrocyte antigens are concerned is that, although immune responses can be mounted, only in extreme circumstances do they result in fetal compromise (e.g. hemolytic disease of the newborn), but they are not thought to be involved in the fundamental issue of fetal survival.

Placental alkaline phosphatase   Although placental alkaline phosphatase has been well characterized, and its polymorphic nature documented, its function is not known. It is found on syncytiotrophoblast but not on other trophoblast cells, and is seen only after the first trimester, thus suggesting that it may not be important in immunoregulation at the maternofetal interface.

Antigens shared by tumors and trophoblast   Certain tumor cells express antigens on the cell surface that are found on trophoblast and embryonic cells. From an oncology point of view, these antigens have been of particular importance as they have in some cases acted as tumor markers and allowed monitoring of disease progression and/or response to treatment. When expressed on trophoblast, the maternal immune system might be expected to respond to them in the same way as the immune system responds to tumor cells. However, therein lies the problem. The malignant tumors that produce oncofetal antigens generally escape surveillance by the immune system, and it is possible that the mechanisms employed by the tumor are similar to those that allow the fetus to escape maternal immunosurveillance. Thus, the mother does not mount a significant response to these antigens.

Complement regulatory proteins on trophoblast   Within such a complex system as the complement system, which acts in a cascade fashion, there is an inherent danger of damage to normal bystander cells, tissues or organs resulting from the fortuitous deposition of activated complement components. Therefore, there is a requirement for stringent control mechanisms. The importance of such control systems is reflected in the fact that there are at least as many proteins involved in essential regulatory function as there are components of the pathways themselves. At the cell surface, at least three membrane-bound proteins – decay-accelerating factor (CD55), membrane co-factor protein (MCP, CD46) and CD59 – have been characterized, and their site of action defined. Perhaps what is likely to turn out to be a very exciting discovery of recent years in reproductive biology is that trophoblast expresses all three proteins in large amounts. Furthermore, they are all expressed where trophoblast surfaces are in contact with maternal blood and tissues, and this expression occurs as early as 6 weeks' gestation. It seems wholly reasonable to assume that the role of these proteins is to protect trophoblast from maternal complement-mediated damage. In addition, it seems that, at the least, part of what used to be regarded as the trophoblast–lymphocyte cross-reactivity (TLX) antigen system is in fact MCP, and this puts paid to the original hypotheses involving cognate recognition of TLX, since a maternal antifetal antibody response to trophoblast MCP could interfere with what is likely to be a most crucial function of this protein on trophoblast, namely protecting trophoblast against damage by maternal complement. The potential involvement of these complement regulatory proteins in pregnancy disorders remains a matter for speculation, but research in this area is as yet in its infancy.

Lack of maternal responsiveness to polymorphic non-MHC antigens to trophoblast   By lacking classical MHC antigens, trophoblast cannot elicit allogeneic responses. In addition, assuming that the phenomenon of MHC restriction applies equally to trophoblast, the absence of classical MHC class I antigens would prevent the co-recognition of any other of the wide-ranging trophoblast cell surface antigens. Thus, none of the trophoblast surface antigens would pose a threat to the survival of trophoblast, while being able to subserve whatever function they are suppose to. The fact that expression of HLA in villous trophoblast cannot be up-regulated by IFN-γ might be an additional failsafe mechanism to prevent maternofetal allorecognition. Complement regulatory proteins protect trophoblast against fortuitous damage by complement.

Immunology of the endometrium and decidua

Cell types in the decidua   Decidualization is the response of the uterine endometrium to the implanting embryo, but as yet the nature or precise source of the stimulus is unknown. The site of implantation where the placenta subsequently forms is called the decidua basalis, while the rest of the decidua is designated decidua parietalis. The decidua contains conventional immunological cell types (lymphocytes, macrophages) and non-conventional immunological cell types, most notably the uterine large granular lymphocytes (U-LGLs). Clearly, immunological responses within the decidua are likely to be crucial, as this is the definitive maternofetal interface. MHC class II+ and CD14+ macrophages, capable of a range of immunological function including antigen presentation, phagocytic activity and secretion of prostaglandins, occur in abundance in the decidua. Conventional T cells are also found, although the proportions of CD4 to CD8 cells appear to be an inverse of the proportions in peripheral blood in that there appear to be relatively more CD8 than CD4 cells. The significance of this is open to conjecture. U-LGLs have attracted a great deal of interest in recent years. They are CD2+, but unlike conventional T cells, they are CD3−. This absence of CD3 implies the absence of the T cell receptor (TcR), suggesting that these cells are not specifically antigen reactive or alloreactive, although they might be activated by another system. They resemble NK cells, but while staining for some NK markers (CD56+, CD57+, HNK-1+), they do not stain for others (CD16−). Functionally, the U-LGLs exhibit NK activity against conventional NK targets, such as the cell line K562. The role of U-LGLs in pregnancy is unknown. Mitotic activity in these cells increases from the proliferative phase through to the late secretory phase of the menstrual cycle, and their numbers increase if pregnancy occurs but decrease if it does not, suggesting a hormonal involvement in the control of their numbers and activity. Conventional NK cells are also found in the decidua, but their activity is less than that in peripheral blood. It is known that in the peripheral blood they decrease in number and activity during pregnancy. Their function in the decidua is unknown, although it has been postulated that they may down-regulate maternal antifetal reactions. Of particular interest has been the report that expression of the HLA-G α-chain protein in HLA-A, -B and -C null cells reduced their susceptibility to NK and T cell-mediated lysis. There is an evolving idea that HLA-G may function on trophoblast as a recognition molecule to prevent lysis by NK cells.

Suppressor activity in the decidua   The concept of suppressor activity in immunological responses remains a controversial issue. This is largely because, although the activity itself is demonstrable, the cells responsible for this effect have not been clearly identified. This suppressive effect can apparently be associated with small non-T, non-B granulocytic lymphocytes, the appearance of which is mediated by a soluble factor that blocks lymphocyte responses. Suppressor cells have been observed in two murine models of pregnancy where resorption of embryos occurs; these are when *Mus caroli* embryos are transferred to *musculus* uteri and in CBA/J C DBA/2 embryos in a CBA/J uterus. In both cases there appears to be a deficiency of the small non-T, non-B granulated suppressor cells. It is claimed that the soluble factor, released by these cells in murine decidua, is related to transforming growth factor-β (TGF-β). A further factor proposed as a mediator of immunosuppressive activity in murine decidua during pregnancy is prostaglandin PGE_2. It has been proposed that NK cells present in decidua become progressively inactivated, and by the 12th day of gestation they are devoid of any killer function against trophoblast cells. It has been suggested that this inactivation comes from local PGE_2 production by decidual cells and decidual macrophages, and is almost completely reversible when prostaglandin synthesis is inhibited in the presence of indomethacin.

Cytokine interactions in the maternofetal relationship   MRL-lpr/lpr homozygous mice have excessive T-cell proliferation along with large placentas that show abnormally high levels of phagocytosis, and the placental phenomena can be reduced to normal by treatment of the pregnant female with anti-T cell antibodies. In normal mice, this treatment reduces placental size and, in some strain combinations, causes fetal resorption. T cells mediate many of their responses via the elaboration of cytokines. Thus, local cytokine production may influence survival and growth of the fetoplacental unit. There is now ample evidence that granulocyte-macrophage colony-stimulating factor (GM-CSF), interleukin-3 (IL-3) and colony-stimulating factor-1 (CSF-1) can promote the growth and/or differentiation of mouse and human trophoblast, and enhance fetal survival when injected into mice prone to foetal resorption. In contrast, other cytokines, such as IL-2, tumor necrosis factor (TNF) and interferon-γ (IFN-γ) appear to have deleterious effects. In addition to cells of the immune system, non-immune components of the reproductive tract, including the uterine epithelium and trophoblast, can also elaborate cytokines. Thus, the concept has emerged that there are beneficial cytokines which can enhance fetal growth and survival, and deleterious cytokines which can compromise pregnancy, and that such cytokines can be elaborated with or without the involvement of the immune system. Studies into the role of cytokines in pregnancy are in their infancy, but it is becoming increasingly clear that many answers will be yielded by these studies.

Maternal immunocompetence during pregnancy

Peter Medawar himself suggested, as of the three potential explanations of the fetal allograft, that the mother might be immunologically indolent or inert during pregnancy. However, as outlined below, the extent of such immunomodulation is limited, and would be unlikely on its own to account for survival of the fetus.

Effect of pregnancy on lymphoid organs

Experiments on laboratory animals have demonstrated clearly that pregnancy affects lymphoid organs. Physiological changes which have been observed in lymphoid organs during both allogeneic and synergeneic murine pregnancy include thymus involution, splenomegaly and changes in humoral and cellular immunity. The thymus is the site of maturation of T lymphocytes, and recent intense research activity has given a great deal of insight into the way in which self-reactive T cells are eliminated during ontogeny. Involution of the thymus during pregnancy has been observed in several species, including man, mouse and rat. The mechanism or nature and indeed the significance of this involution remains somewhat unclear. The involution is thought to be due to an exodus of small lymphocytes from the thymic cortex in response to steroid hormones. This involution is a non-specific effect of pregnancy, occurring in both allogeneic and synergeneic pregnancy, and the cellularity of the thymus is thought to return to normal after the period of lactation. Enlargement of the spleen has been reported in human pregnancy. In murine studies, splenomegaly has been clearly documented; it reaches its maximal size at midgestation, returning to normal at about 20 days postpartum. In this model, the rate of erythropoiesis in the spleen changes during pregnancy, and it would seem that antigens, estrogen and progesterone as well as erythropoietin affect this rate.

Estrogen appears to stimulate the production of large and medium erythrocytes in the spleen. The enlargement of the spleen is accompanied by an increase in the numbers of immunoglobulin-producing cells. Teleologically, this increase makes sense, since the increase in circulating maternal immunoglobulin will make extra immunoglobulins available for passive transfer to the fetus. Lymph node changes have been studied in humans, and there is histological evidence of a diminution in the germinal centers at term in the para-aortic lymph nodes which drain the uterus. Similar changes have been found in murine studies. The stimulus that produces the increase in lymph nodes is not known, but may be of fetal origin, since removal of the fetus without removing the placenta abrogates the observed increase.

Maternal responses to infection in pregnancy

Perhaps influenced by the general assumption that there must be some form of immunosuppression in the mother to allow for the survival of the fetal semiallograft, it has long been assumed that pregnancy increases women's susceptibility to infections. Indeed, there are data suggesting an increase in the clinical severity of certain infections when they are newly acquired in pregnancy. Other infections, such as leprosy, tend to be more severe in late pregnancy, and the incidence of listeriosis is generally increased. Latent viral infections may be reactivated in pregnancy. However, the vast majority of women experience healthy, infection-free pregnancies, and the

35

consensus of opinion is therefore that the maternal immune responses to infection during pregnancy are adequate.

Humoral and cell-mediated responses to conventional antigens

Responses to both novel and recall conventional antigens have been studied in pregnant women. There is general acceptance that both humoral and cellular responses are not significantly different from those in non-pregnant women.

T and B cell subpopulations in pregnancy

Since the numbers and relative ratios of circulating immune cells are likely to reflect overall immunocompetence, the effects of pregnancy on these parameters have been widely studied. Some studies have found significant changes while others have not. However, the general consensus of opinion is that, if indeed there are changes in T and B cell numbers and ratios in pregnancy, these changes are not biologically relevant to any putative immunodeficiency of pregnancy.

Studies of lymphocyte function have also generated conflicting data, some groups reporting depression of responses to mitogens, while other groups have failed to corroborate these findings. More importantly, whether these *in vitro* findings can be extrapolated to the situation *in vivo* is doubtful.

Natural killer cells in pregnancy

NK cells are capable of killing some tumor cells spontaneously without prior sensitization. They do not seem to have immunological memory and can lyse cells that are syngeneic, allogeneic or xenogeneic to the NK cell donor. During human pregnancy, NK activity decreases from 16 weeks until term, returning to control levels after delivery. Studies have shown that, in addition to a decrease in NK cell numbers during pregnancy, the cells which remain have less lytic activity. However, as yet the role of this change in number and activity of peripheral NK cells in the success or otherwise of pregnancy is not known. In addition, the factors that directly cause this change have yet to be elucidated. It is thought that NK cells may be suppressed *in vivo* by prostaglandins released by macrophages, and this may be especially true for the U-LGLs in the decidua. Of particular interest in this regard has been the observation that the administration of indomethacin *in vitro* blocks NK activity and *in vivo* produces abortion in more than 70% of susceptible mouse strains. Newer ideas on a possible role for NK cells in recurrent miscarriage are discussed in Chapter 3.1.

Candidate immunosuppressor factors in pregnancy

Pregnancy is accompanied by profound changes in the hormonal milieu, including steroid hormones, trophoblast-derived molecules such as chorionic gonadotropins and α-fetoprotein (AFP). It is evident that some hormones, especially the steroids, modulate the immune response in pregnancy; the classic observations of Hench on the amelioration of rheumatoid arthritis in pregnancy subsequently led to the use of steroids in the treatment of this condition and to Hench being award the Nobel Prize. The mechanism of action of cortisone remains an enigma, and although among animals rodents are particularly susceptible to the immunosuppressive effects of steroids, humans appear to be more resistant. Despite their widespread use in the suppression of autoimmune disease, there is no evidence to suggest that the elevated levels of steroids seen in pregnancy significantly suppress the mother's overall immune response. Of the sex steroids, progesterone has been shown to depress the mixed lymphocyte reaction (MLR) in humans, but only at high concentrations equivalent to those reached in the later stages of pregnancy, so that it is difficult to extrapolate the *in vitro* findings to the situation *in vivo*. AFP, a major pregnancy hormone, has been shown to inhibit both the MLR and mitogen responses in mouse and human, but in both situations the degree of immunosuppression did not correlate with the concentration of AFP, and the influence of contaminants could not be excluded. While early work suggested that human chorionic gonadotropin might be a powerful immunosuppressant, subsequent work suggested that the suppressive effects were again due to contaminants. A whole range of other pregnancy-associated proteins have been studied, but the data have remained inconclusive and often contradictory between different centers. Thus, many of the candidate immunosuppressor factors in pregnancy do indeed possess immunosuppressive properties *in vitro*, but whether these are relevant to survival of the fetal semiallograft is doubtful.

Concluding remarks on maternal immunocompetence in pregnancy

There is ample evidence for some degree of diminution in the maternal immune response in pregnancy, and hormones, steroids and other factors produced in abundance in pregnancy may account for this observation. However, in general, women remain sufficiently immunocompetent during pregnancy to remain healthy, and the degree of immunodepression observed cannot account for the failure to eradicate as powerful a stimulus as an allograft. While fetal survival could largely be based on an effective physical barrier which, on the one hand, does not express classical HLA antigens yet, on the other, expresses large amounts of complement regulatory proteins, it is clear that, throughout evolution, extensive 'failsafe' mechanisms have evolved in parallel with the evolution of complex biological systems. Reproduction is central to continuation of the species, and it is therefore not surprising that elaborate mechanisms have evolved to prevent deleterious maternal immunological responses against the fetus. Thus, all the other immune down-regulatory phenomena observed within the mother, which by themselves cannot explain the survival of the fetal semiallograft, could be viewed as acting synergistically with the central mechanism of an immunologically inert trophoblast, to ensure the continuation of the species. In this way, the immune system allows the propagation of the species without leaving the body open to attack by exogenous pathogens.

Activation of the maternal innate immune system in pregnancy: a novel concept

As long ago as the mid-to-late 1970s it was recognized that normal pregnancy was associated with markers of systemic inflammation. Thus, it has long been known that leukocytosis occurs in normal pregnancy, and that the clotting system is also activated in normal pregnancy. However, it was not until the late 1990s that it became evident that there were strong systemic inflammatory changes in normal pregnancy, readily detectable in the third trimester, but possibly being initiated in the first or second trimester. Significant changes relative to normal non-pregnant women include evidence of the following:

- Complement activation, with a rise in levels of factors C1q, C3, C4, C4d

- Leukocytosis – increase in absolute numbers of monocytes and granulocytes

- Increased leukocyte activation – as evidenced by activation markers and phago-cytosis

- Activation of the clotting system and increase in other acute-phase proteins

- Platelet activation

- Increase in markers of oxidative stress, either generated *de novo* or as part of the systemic inflammatory response

- Markers of endothelial cell activation, including plasminogen activator inhibitor-1, endothelin and vascular endothelial growth factor

A consistent and opposite finding with regard to the activation of the innate immune system is that NK cell numbers, cytotoxic activity and production of IFN-γ are decreased.

It is not known what activates the innate immune system. It is well established that in normal pregnancy the placenta sheds both particulate and soluble products (syncytiotrophoblast membrane fragments (STBMs), fetal DNA, other cellular components and products of apoptosis). It has been suggested that these placental products may be the stimulus to the innate system, and indeed may differentially interact with the innate and adaptive systems, causing suppression of the latter, while stimulating the former. A form of 'cascade reaction' might occur: monocytes might be the first and direct target of stimulation by the placental products, and they in turn might release proinflammatory substances including cytokines, lipids, enzymes and free radicals, which then amplify the systemic inflammatory response. There is *in vitro* evidence of monocyte activation by STBMs, and a whole range of other pregnancy-related circulating factors have been shown to activate monocytes on the one hand, while suppressing lymphocytes on the other. These include:

- STBMs
- Human placental lactogen
- Human chorionic gonadotropin
- Corticotropin releasing hormone
- Progesterone
- Vascular endothelial growth factor

The significance of the activation of the innate system for pregnancy outcome is unknown. It has been speculated that the activation might play a role in protection against infection, but there is no clear indication that the pregnant woman would be more susceptible to infection were the innate system to function in the same way as in the non-pregnant state. Indeed, an activated innate system might contribute to increased severity of some maternal infections (see Chapter 5 on 'Immunopathology'). Could activation of the innate system be simply an epiphenomenon?

Whatever the real significance of this activation, it has received particular attention in recent years for two reasons:

Recurrent miscarriage   In normal pregnancy, in the face of systemic activation of the innate immune system, not only are NK cells (a major component of the innate system) reduced in absolute numbers, but their cytotoxic activity and their production of IFN-γ are also reduced. These observations become significant in the light of recent reports which suggest that a subpopulation of women with recurrent miscarriage (and/or subfertility) have elevated NK cell numbers and activity in peripheral blood and/or in the decidua, and that these NK cells may be contributing to the clinical problem. This issue is discussed in detail in Chapter 3.1.

Pre-eclampsia   A rather attractive hypothesis has been proffered in recent years which suggests that pre-eclampsia is really no more than an exaggeration of the normal innate systemic inflammatory response, the exaggeration causing decompensation in one or another system and leading to features of the pre-eclampsia syndrome. This concept is further discussed in Chapter 3.2

Maternal immune responses to fetal antigens

There is now ample evidence that the mother makes both humoral and cellular immune responses to fetal antigens. In this section, the mechanisms for sensitizing the mother, and the nature and the significance of the immune responses, are reviewed.

Maternal sensitization to fetal antigens

There is irrefutable evidence that at least some, if not all, pregnant women make demonstrable responses to fetal antigens, especially paternally derived MHC antigens. It is interesting to speculate how the mother comes into contact with these antigens. The molecular basis of allorecognition of foreign MHC antigens is thought to be cross-reactivity by antigen-specific, self-MHC-restricted, T cells. Allorecognition is thus structurally heterogeneous and influenced by the disparity between the MHC antigens of the responder and the stimulator. In disparate responder–stimulator combinations the alloresponse may be directed against residues on the MHC molecule itself, while in closely related combinations alloreactive T cells might recognize epitopes of endogenous peptides that are displayed by stimulator but not by responder MHC molecules, seen in a self-restricted vigor of alloresponses and the widely reported unusually high precursor frequency of alloreactive T cells. It was stated earlier that there is no vascular continuity between the maternal and fetal compartments, and that fetally derived tissue (trophoblast) in direct contact with the maternal immune system is either devoid of MHC antigens, or expresses the monomorphic HLA-G. It has been argued that MHC-bearing fetal cells routinely enter the maternal circulation, and indeed a great deal of research effort has been expended on developing prenatal diagnostic techniques based on isolating these fetal cells from the peripheral blood of pregnant women. However, the passage of fetal cells into the maternal circulation is likely to be a sporadic event due to maternofetal hemorrhage, rather than a facilitated process. This would explain why only a proportion of women develop antibodies to paternal HLA, and why the incidence of these antibodies appears to increase with increasing gestation and parity.

Alloantibody responses

The presence of alloantibodies in pregnancy sera was described independently by two groups. The technique used by both groups demonstrated leukoagglutinating antibodies, but subsequent use of complement-dependent techniques showed the presence of leukocytoxic antibodies (LCAs). It is now well established that LCAs are directed to paternal, rather than third-party, antigens, that the incidence of LCAs increases with increasing parity, that the frequency of LCA occurrence dips in the last trimester, that the LCAs may be immunoglobulin G (IgG) as well as IgM and that the placenta acts as a sink for antiallotypic antibodies, and that these antibodies can be eluted from this placental sink. Even among multiparas some women never make these antibodies, and all studies to date show that no more than 50% of multiparas have these antibodies. The reason for the lack of response is unknown, but it may be that techniques of detection are not sufficiently sensitive, or the LCAs may be made but may be blocked by anti-idiotypes (see below), or these women may be true non-responders, a phenomenon seen in some mice. The role of anti-HLA antibodies in nature is not known. However, they do not seem to be essential for the success of pregnancy.

Mixed lymphocyte reaction-blocking antibodies

It has been suggested that mixed lymphocyte reaction (MLR) inhibition might be a more sensitive assay than LCA activity for detecting antipaternal antibodies, for in studies of MLR-blocking activity there were fewer sera with LCA activity than MLR-inhibiting sera. MLR inhibition tends to be specific, and directed at paternal rather than maternal stimulators, although inhibition of third-party stimulators may also occur. The significance of MLR inhibition remains unclear. It could be speculated that, since the response is directed at paternal HLA antigens, their role *in vivo* is to mask paternally derived fetal HLA antigens and thereby prevent recognition by maternal alloreactive T cells. However, the fact that MLR inhibition or LCAs are not universal phenomena would tend to militate against their having such a fundamental role.

Anti-idiotypic antibodies

The theory of idiotype and anti-idiotype networks lends itself well to hypotheses in pregnancy, but experiments in this field are difficult to conduct and few laboratories have explored this area. Theoretical considerations are nevertheless fascinating. The evidence from both *in vivo* and *in vitro* observations above shows that the mother can mount anti-HLA responses to paternally derived fetal antigens. However, such responses are potentially harmful, so the mother may well need to mount another response to block the first. In idiotype terminology, the first response produces (anti-HLA) antibody-1, the idiotype, and the second produces (anti-anti-HLA antibody) the anti-idiotype. Some investigators have proposed that this explains the absence of LCAs or MLR-blocking activity in the sera of some multiparas – that they are in fact present but are masked by anti-idiotypic antibodies. The hypothesis is not limited to antibody–antibody responses, but can also be extended to T cell responses. If the TcR on maternal T cell clones is regarded as the idiotype, the mother might produce antibodies to this TcR, the anti-idiotype, and experimental evidence has been

41

reported to support this view. In this study, antipaternal alloreactive T cell clones were established. IgG from the mother's pregnancy reacted with these clones, but not with T cell clones to other unrelated HLA. An MLR between these clones (responders) and paternal cells could be blocked by maternal serum, but not when the responders were control T cell clones. Interestingly, high concentrations of the antigen-binding$_2$ fragment (Fab$_2$) of her IgG, bound to a paternal-specific T cell clone, blocked its cytolytic activity and stimulated the clone to proliferate.

Antibodies to trophoblast and placental antigens

Antibodies, shown by adsorption studies not to be directed at the HLA system, but binding to trophoblast, have been reported. Some of the antibody occurs in the form of immune complexes, and a degree of specificity has been reported, suggesting that perhaps there may be an as yet undefined polymorphic system, distinct from MHC, within trophoblast. However, the explanation may be really quite simple: trophoblast possesses Fc (crystallizable fragment) receptors of IgG, and therefore binding of immunoglobulins to trophoblast does not necessarily mean that the Fab fragments are binding to epitopes on trophoblast antigens. The nature, incidence, specificity and possible significance of antitrophoblast antibodies remains to be unraveled.

Antibodies to erythrocyte antigens

Erythrocytes display a wide range of polymorphic antigenic systems to which the maternal immune system can mount a response. However, although such responses, especially responses involving the rhesus antigens, can compromise the fetus, they are not generally regarded as playing a crucial role in the fundamental question of the immunological paradox. They are therefore not discussed any further here: suffice it to acknowledge their occurrence.

T cell responses

Since T cells are thought to be the major effector cells in allograft rejection, they have been an obvious target of investigation with respect to their behavior in pregnancy. Studies of alloreactive responses are made particularly difficult by a pre-existing high precursor frequency of alloreactive cells, even in the absence of prior exposure to alloantigen.

In vivo cell-mediated immune responses

There are obvious ethical constraints to studying cell-mediated immune (CMI) responses to allografts in pregnant women. Most of the available data are therefore based on animal work. The essential experiments have sought to establish whether pre-pregnancy sensitization of a mother to paternal and fetal alloantigens would affect subsequent pregnancies, using sensitization techniques that are known to accelerate subsequent graft rejection. Such sensitization did not affect subsequent pregnancies. These findings parallel the observation in humans that the formation of LCAs (evidence of allosensitization) does not appear to affect subsequent pregnancies.

In vitro cell-mediated immune responses

In humans, as in other animal models, CMI responses to paternal or fetal antigens have been studied indirectly *in vitro* by means of MLR and cytotoxic T lymphocyte (CTL) assays. Some studies have reported that the antipaternal MLR increased as pregnancy advanced, but other studies could find neither an anamnesic MLR in parous women nor significant CTL responses to paternal MHC-bearing cells. In more recent studies using the sensitive and quantitative technique of limited dilution analysis, other researchers have demonstrated the presence of wide ranges of antipaternal cytotoxic T cells in the peripheral blood of both primiparas and multiparas, but that the frequencies of these cells did not alter throughout pregnancy. Thus, the consensus of opinion is that pregnancy is not accompanied by increased T cell reactivity to fetal antigens, and that when this does occur, it does not prejudice pregnancy outcome.

Graft versus host disease in nature

Owing to a lack of vascular continuity between the maternal and fetal compartments, in normal pregnancy, no exchange of cellular material occurs. However, the trophoblast is a minimal barrier, and might be expected to be breached from time to time. Fetal cells entering the maternal circulation might expect to be destroyed, and the worst they could do is elicit formation of antipaternal cytotoxic antibody. The effect of immunocompetent maternal cells entering the fetal compartment would, however, create the possibility of the development of graft versus host disease (GvHD), since the fetus may express paternally derived HLA, and its own immune system may be too immature to destroy the maternal cells. It is now clear that what was at one time regarded as a purely theoretical hazard of pregnancy does indeed occur in nature. The first case report described XX/XY lymphoid chimerism in an infant with an immunodeficiency syndrome, and this was interpreted as a case of GvHD with secondary immunological failure. Other cases followed. It is well recognized that ABO compatibility between mother and fetus exacerbates rhesus isoimmunization, since any fetal red cells entering the maternal circulation tend to persist longer. An analogous situation might be expected in maternofetal GvHD: the T cells from a mother homozygous at one or more HLA loci would be able to react against paternally derived HLA antigens on the fetus but the fetus would not react against the maternal T cells because the homozygous HLA gene products will be seen as self. Reports do indeed exist of increased HLA-DR compatibility between mother and child in severe combined immunodeficiency (SCID) and other neonatal hematopoietic diseases, and this suggests that instances of SCID where there is no clear autosomal recessive inheritance might represent the outcome of GvHD.

Immunology has long been criticized for being largely theoretical and contributing little to practical aspects of clinical practice. For example, some would contend that the major advances in transplantation have not come from immunology, but from improved immunosuppressive therapy and surgical skill. However, there are interesting, if anecdotal, examples of immunologic engineering in the literature. To eliminate maternal cells (graft 1) causing GvHD in a child with SCID, a bone marrow graft (graft 2) from an HLA-identical sibling was given to the SCID child. There was a temporary exacerbation of the GvHD, but the graft-versus-graft situation created resulted in the formation of CTLs which were able to eliminate the maternal T cells (graft 1).

2.2 Fetal and neonatal immunology

During the intrauterine period and at the time of birth, the fetus and neonate are susceptible to both bacterial and viral infections. The fetus is surrounded by a relatively stagnant but nutrient-rich pool of amniotic fluid, which could promote bacterial infection, while it can be expected that its immunity, along with all its other systems, is immature and would be largely ineffective against most viral infections. Infections of the fetus are in reality relatively rare, and those in the neonatal period are usually self-limiting or readily overcome. All of this is largely thanks to the mother, who provides a highly effective physical and passive immunological protective barrier to both the fetus and the neonate. The immune system also starts to develop in early gestation, but is still significantly immature even at term delivery. Therefore the extent and nature of the infectious risks posed by bacteria and viruses is dependent upon the extent to which passive immunity has been transferred, and the immune maturity of the fetus/neonate (and therefore the gestation at birth). Two main issues are therefore addressed in this brief chapter, namely placental transfer of IgG, and the development of the fetal immune system.

PLACENTAL TRANSFER OF IMMUNOGLOBULIN G

Passive transfer of IgG from the maternal into the fetal compartment begins at about 12 weeks' gestation, but in fact most of the maternal immunoglobulin is transferred after 32 weeks of intrauterine life (Figure 2.3). Extremely premature babies, therefore, lack circulating maternal IgG at birth and are susceptible to infection. Infants with poor fetal growth also have lower levels of IgG at birth, due to poor placental transfer. IgG is transferred by means of specific receptors on the trophoblast for the Fc (crystallizable fragment) region of IgG.

Owing to transfer of IgG from the mother, the full-term baby has serum levels of IgG equivalent to those of the mother. However, the levels fall quite dramatically as there is little active neonatal synthesis of IgG or IgA at this stage. The half-life of IgG is 3–4 weeks, and the period between 3 and 6 months is a phase of relative immunoglobulin deficiency ('physiological trough'). This is associated with increasing expression of CD40 ligand on T cells, which is initially low at birth. Furthermore, the immaturity of B cells at birth, i.e. their CD5+ nature, may result in low-affinity antibody protection. Maturation of antibody production, including isotype switching to IgG and IgA, as well as to high affinity, depends on the interaction of CD40 ligand and B cells, and is accomplished by 2 months of age when routine immunizations with protein antigens begin. The serum IgG level rises to reach normal levels by the age of 2 years (Figure 2.3), by which time antibodies to carbohydrate antigens are produced too.

There are instances in which administration of exogenous immunoglobulin might be beneficial to the neonate. This is the case in babies born to mothers who

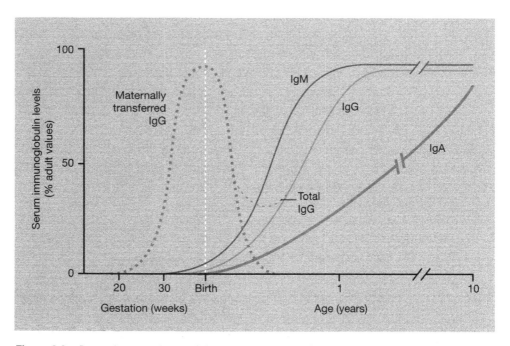

Figure 2.3 Serum immunoglobulin (Ig) levels and age. Maximal transfer of immunoglobulins from mother to fetus occurs after 32 weeks of gestation, thus explaining why very premature babies do not enjoy maternally derived protection against infection. Maternally derived IgG has mostly disappeared by 6 months. As the neonate actively synthesizes IgG the level slowly rises, but a physiological 'trough' of serum IgG is seen between 3 and 6 months. Adapted from Chapel H *et al*. Essentials of Clinical Immunology, 4th edn. Blackwell Science, 1999: 308

are hepatitis B surface-antigen-positive, and in the USA, replacement immuno-globulin is more often administered, especially in very-low-birth-weight infants who are frequently subjected to invasive procedures. In this group, intravenous immunoglobulin (IVIG) infusions have been shown to reduce late-onset infections in placebo-controlled studies. IVIG is not used routinely in the UK, since the rate of serious late-onset infections is less than 1%, probably due to avoidance of invasive procedures whenever possible. Replacement immunoglobulin is not needed in the physiological trough unless the child suffers from serious recurrent infections, which are not preventable with prophylactic antibiotics.

DEVELOPMENT OF CELLULAR IMMUNE RESPONSIVENESS IN THE FETUS

Table 2.1 charts what is currently known about cellular immune development in the fetus. This illustrates that at least partial immunocompetence develops early in intrauterine life, with the fetus being able to produce IgM antibodies as early as 11 weeks' gestation in response to intrauterine infection with rubella virus. However, T cell development is slow, and this may account for the particular susceptibility of the fetus to viruses and intracellular bacteria. Although T cells are detectable early in gestational life, their functional capacity develops late, is still reduced at birth, but increases in early life to reach adult levels in the first 2 months.

At birth, although CD4+ cells are high and IL-2 production is normal, INF-γ and Th2 cytokine production is low and cytotoxic T cell function is only one-third of that of adults. Natural killer cell activity is 50% of adult levels too. These findings may account for the severity of neonatal infections with herpes simplex virus, cytomegalovirus, *Listeria* and *Toxoplasma*. *Listeria*, a facultative intracellular bacterium, is killed as a result of CD8+ cytotoxic T cells recognizing listerial antigen in the context of MHC class I antigens on the surface of the infected histiocyte or hepatocyte. Secretion of tumor necrosis factor (TNF) is also crucial, since the absence of TNF receptors on the host cell in the mouse model (TNF receptor knock-out mouse) results in overwhelming infection. With reduced cytotoxic T cells and T_{h1} cytokine production, the fetus is more susceptible than the mother.

The fetus is protected against bacterial infection by active transfer of maternal IgG across the placenta as described above. Fortunately, neutrophil leukocytes and macrophages are fully competent and plentiful in the circulation within a few days of birth.

Table 2.1   Development of immune responsiveness in the fetus. Adapted from Chapel H *et al*. Essentials of Clinical Immunology, 4th edn. Blackwell Science, 1999: 307

Gestational age (weeks)	Immune development
4	blood center with macrophages in the yolk sac
6	complement synthesis detected
6	NK cells present in liver
6–7	thymic epithelium develops
7	lymphocytes and macrophages in blood
7–9	lymphocytes in thymus: CD3+, 4+, 8+, TCR+
11	serum IgM detectable in infection (e.g. rubella)
	mitogen responsiveness of thymocytes
12–14	neutrophil leucocytes in blood
13	B cells in bone marrow
14	mitogen responsiveness of peripheral lymphocytes
17	endogenous IgG in serum – in infection only
20	alloreactivity detected
Term	B cells
	normal numbers but immature, i.e. CD5+
	antibodies
	IgM to proteins but not to carbohydrate antigens
	complement
	classical 90%, alternative 60% adult levels
	C8 and C9 only 20% of adult levels
	T cells
	higher numbers than adult levels but immature
	cytokines
	IL-2 production normal
	IFN-γ only 20% of adult levels
	Th2 cytokines very low
	activity
	cytotoxic T cells only 30–60% of adult levels
	NK cell activity only 50% of adult levels

NK, natural killer; IL-2, interleukin 2; IFN-γ, interferon-γ

IMMUNOPATHOLOGY INVOLVING THE FETUS/NEONATE

Hemolytic disease of the newborn

Adaptive immune responses evolved to protect vertebrate species against the world of micro-organisms. However, anything discerned as 'non-self' may become a target of such responses, which can also be directed at molecular differences between individuals within a species. An antibody directed against an antigenic determinant

Table 2.2 ABO blood group typing and cross-matching for blood transfusion. Hemoagglutination is used to type blood groups and match compatible donors and recipients for blood transfusions. Common Gram-negative bacterial surface antigens that are similar or identical to blood group antigens, stimulate the formation of antibodies to these antigens in individuals who do not bear the corresponding antigen on their own red blood cells; thus, type O individuals who lack A and B, have both anti-A and anti-B antibodies, whereas type AB individuals have neither. The pattern of agglutination of the red blood cells of a transfusion donor or recipient with anti-A and anti-B antibodies reveals the individual's ABO blood group. Before transfusion, the serum of the recipient is also tested for antibodies that agglutinate the red blood cells of a donor, and vice versa, a procedure called a cross-match, which may detect potentially harmful antibodies to other blood groups that are not part of the ABO system

Blood group	Antigens expressed in red blood cells	Antibodies produced in serum	Compatible blood type
O*	NONE	anti-A anti-B	ONLY 'O' type blood
A	'A' antigen	anti-B	'O' and 'A' type blood
B	'B' antigen	anti-A	'O' and 'B' type blood
AB†	'A' and 'B' antigens	NONE	'O', 'A', 'B' and 'AB' type blood

*Blood group O, 'universal donor'; †blood group AB, 'universal recipient'

present In some members of a species but not in others is said to show polymorphic variation, and antibodies directed against such determinants are called alloantibodies. Perhaps the best known alloantibodies are those that are used to determine our blood groups. Individuals who have red cells of type A have alloantibodies that react with the red cells of individuals who are type B and vice versa. Individuals who have red blood cells of type AB have no alloantibodies and those with type O red blood cells have antibodies to both A and B red blood cells (Table 2.2). These alloantibodies arise from the fact that the capsules of Gram-negative bacteria, which inhabit our gut, bear antigens that stimulate antibodies that cross-react with the carbohydrate antigens of the ABO blood groups. A serious problem is posed frequently by alloantibodies induced by a fetus in the pregnant mother. Alloimmunization most often results from rhesus incompatibility between mother and fetus. Approximately 13% of women are rhesus-negative; that is, their red blood cells do not bear the rhesus antigen. A woman who is rhesus-negative has an 87% chance of marrying a rhesus-positive man and their chances of having a rhesus-positive baby are very high. Not infrequently, during delivery of the new born, some blood escapes from the fetal circulation into the maternal circulation and the mother develops alloantibodies to the rhesus antigen as a result. During a subsequent pregnancy with a rhesus-positive fetus, the maternal IgG alloantibodies cross the placenta and cause hemolysis of the fetal red cells. The consequence of this can be very grave and result in fetal death or severe damage to the newborn infant.

The rhesus antigenic determinants are spaced far apart on the red cell surface. As a consequence, IgG antibodies to the rhesus antigen do not fix complement and, therefore, do not hemolyse red blood cells *in vitro*. For reasons that are less well understood, IgG antibodies to the rhesus antigen do not agglutinate rhesus-positive red blood cells. Because of this it was very difficult to detect rhesus antibodies until Professor Robin Coombs at the University of Cambridge devised a solution to the problem by developing antibodies against human immunoglobulin. He showed that rhesus-positive red blood cells coated with IgG anti-rhesus antibodies could be taken from a fetus and agglutinated by antibodies to IgG. Furthermore, he showed that when the serum of an alloimmunized woman was incubated with rhesus-positive red blood cells, these red blood cells could then be agglutinated by antibody to IgG (Figure 2.4). The former is called the direct Coombs' test, and the latter the indirect Coombs' test. This application of immunology to a vexing clinical problem led ultimately to a treatment and prevention of the problem.

Although hemolytic disease of the newborn is most commonly the result of alloimmunization with rhesus antigen, other red blood cell alloantigens, such as Louis, Kell, Duffy, Kidd, Luleran and still others, may cause alloimmunization. In any case, the maternal IgG antibodies cross the placenta in increasing amounts during the second trimester of pregnancy and hemolyse the fetal red blood cells. The resulting anemia may become so severe that, if untreated, the fetus goes into heart failure and develops massive edema; this is called hydrops fetalis and results in fetal death. The risk of fetal development of hydrops rises from 10% when the indirect Coombs' titer of the mother is $1:16$, to 75% when the maternal titer is $1:128$. If the anemia is not so severe as to cause hydrops, the affected infant at birth is still massively hemolysing red blood cells. There is now a need for the newborn to dispose of the heme breakdown pigments rapidly because an excessive accumulation of bilirubin results in the deposition of this pigment in the brain, and severe neurological impairment. In response to the profound anemia, the number of red cell progenitors (erythroblasts) in the spleen, liver and bone marrow expands rapidly; for this reason, hemolytic disease of the newborn has also been called erythroblastosis fetalis.

The extent of hemolysis can be determined easily by obtaining amniotic fluid into which the fetus commences to urinate by 20 weeks of gestation. The quantity of bilirubin excreted into the amniotic fluid correlates with the amount of hemolysis in the fetus. Second, the fetus can be followed by ultrasonography for the development

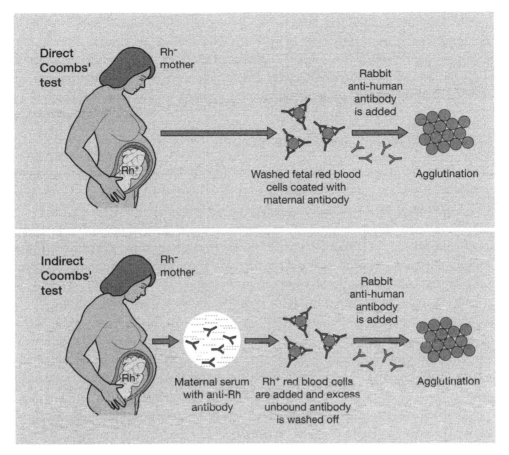

Figure 2.4 The Coombs' direct and indirect antiglobulin test for antibody to red blood cell antigens. A rhesus-negative mother of a rhesus-positive fetus can become immunized to fetal red blood cells that enter the maternal circulation at the time of delivery. In a subsequent pregnancy with a rhesus-positive fetus, IgG anti-rhesus antibodies can cross the placenta and damage the fetal red blood cells. In contrast to anti-rhesus antibodies, anti-ABO antibodies are of the IgM isotype and cannot cross the placenta, and so do not cause harm. Anti-rhesus antibodies do not agglutinate red blood cells, but their presence can be shown by washing the fetal red blood cells and then adding antibody to human immunoglobulin, which agglutinates the antibody-coated cells. The washing removes unrelated immunoglobulins that would otherwise react with the anti-human immunoglobulin antibody. Anti-rhesus antibodies can be detected in the mother's serum in an indirect Coombs' test, the serum is incubated with rhesus-positive red blood cells, and once the antibody binds, the red cells are treated as in the direct Coombs' test

of hydrops. Third, the degree of anemia can be ascertained directly, but with some difficulty, by obtaining a sample of blood from the umbilical vein, a procedure called cord centesis and now routinely performed in most fetal medicine units.

It has become possible in the past few decades to eliminate to a very great extent hemolytic disease of the newborn. All rhesus-negative women are given 300 μg of purified immunoglobulin specific for the rhesus antigen (Rhogam) at 28 weeks of gestation and again within 72 h of delivery. The amount of Rhogam in one vial (300 µg) is sufficient to neutralize 30 ml of fetal blood in the maternal circulation. This procedure fails to prevent alloimmunization in 0.1% of rhesus-negative women, and this must explain the failure to completely eradicate the disease.

Alloimmune thrombocytopenic purpura

Transfer of fetal platelets across the placenta may elicit a maternal antifetal platelet response. If the resultant antibodies are of the IgG variety, they may cross the placenta and result in alloimmune neonatal thrombocytopenic purpura (AITP). This condition is not as rare as previously thought, and is estimated to occur in 1 : 1000 births. However, the antigen to which these antibodies are directed (HPA-1A) is common in the general population, and in practice the majority of mothers are positive for the antigen and do not produce antibodies.

AITP should be distinguished from idiopathic thrombocytopenic purpura (ITP), in which the mother has circulating antibodies to her own platelets. Since these antibodies tend to be of the IgG variety, they can cross the placenta and induce neonatal thrombocytopenia in 50% of infants. Testing of the mother's and the baby's platelets will show whether the antibody is present on platelets from both individuals (due to ITP) or only in the neonate (due to alloimmunization).

A similar mechanism has been detected in which antineutrophil antibodies cause neonatal neutropenia, but this is extremely rare.

2.3 Immunological advantages of breast-feeding

INTRODUCTION

Modern technology enables the artificial replication of all the nutritional components of human breast milk, but it is not possible (yet) to recreate those components
that render human milk vastly superior to any artificial feed: at an emotional level,
the bonding that breast-feeding promotes; and at an immunological level, the
protective factors contributing to the deficient mucosal immune system of the
neonate. The mammary gland functions as part of the common mucosal immune
system, contributing to the neonate antibodies, cells and a whole host of other
protective factors in milk. Thus, pregnant women and new mothers are bombarded
with literature that promotes breast-feeding, and maternity units are given World
Health Organization (WHO) awards for achieving breast-feeding targets! Good
research abounds that demonstrates protective effects of breast-feeding against a
wide range of infections, such as cholera, giardiasis, salmonellosis and shigellosis (but
not the human immunodeficiency virus). Breast-fed infants are less frequently
hospitalized in the first 3 months of life; and are protected against atopic diseases
such as asthma. This chapter explores the immunological protective role of breast-
feeding (Figure 2.5).

THE MAMMARY GLAND PARTICIPATES IN THE COMMON MUCOSAL IMMUNE SYSTEM

Mucosal sites, such as the gastrointestinal tract, genital tract, salivary gland and the
respiratory system, are part of a common mucosal immune system, which refers to
the linking of lymphocytes present at mucosal surfaces (see Chapter 1) to lympho-

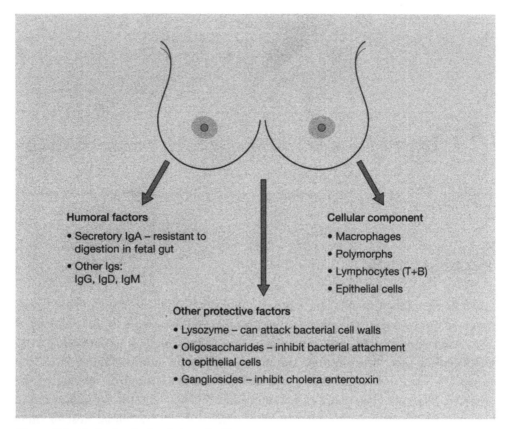

Figure 2.5   Protective factors in breast milk

cytes found in subepithelial surfaces of other mucosal sites. The mammary gland in lactating women is part of this common mucosal immune system. Lymphocytes may be activated by antigens at one mucosal site and selectively home to other mucosal sites. For example, in pregnant women, infection with *Salmonella typhi mourium* results in high levels of salmonella-specific IgA agglutinins in colostrum, while injection of non-pathogenic *Escherichia coli* stimulates colostral antibody formation. In the natural setting, during the respiratory syncytial virus (RSV) season, there is a boosting of the RSV-specific IgA in lactating women. These observations clearly link the gastrointestinal tract, respiratory tract and mammary gland mucosal immune systems in lactating women. The underlying mechanisms involved are still poorly understood, but evidence suggests specific, directed homing of both T and B cells to the mammary glands.

HUMORAL IMMUNOLOGICAL FACTORS IN COLOSTRUM/BREAST MILK

Immunoglobulins found in human milk include IgG, IgD and IgM, but the principal immunoglobulin of human milk is secretory IgA (SIgA), in keeping with the predominance of IgA at other mucosal surfaces. There are two key properties of SIgA with regard to its role in mucosal immunity: first, the secretory component, a glycoprotein transporter receptor, allows transportation across the glandular epithelium; and second, the SIgA is resistant to proteolytic digestion, protecting the IgA against digestion in the infant's gastrointestinal tract. It is interesting to note that the actual total SIgA ingested by infants remains constant (0.5–0.6 g per day) for the first 4 months of lactation, although the concentration of SIgA falls as the volume of milk expands. The individual immunoglobulin subclasses also differ in concentration from those found in serum, but the significance is unclear. For example, while in serum IgG1 is highest in concentration, IgG4 is found in higher concentrations in breast milk. The immunoglobulins in milk presumably provide passive immunity for the infant, whose mucosal immune system is deficient in the first weeks of life.

CELLULAR IMMUNOLOGICAL COMPONENTS IN COLOSTRUM/BREAST MILK

Cells found in human colostrum/milk include macrophages, polymorphs, lymphocytes and epithelial cells, but the relative proportions of these cells change dramatically with time. While macrophages predominate in the first 2 weeks, and there are few epithelial cells, by the end of 1 month epithelial cells predominate. Lymphocytes contribute a small, fairly constant proportion (about 5–7%) through the first 2 months. Research into the functional capabilities of the cellular components has yielded intriguing results. The macrophages display normal phagocytic activity, except for *Candida albicans*, while polymorphs seem to have decreased phagocytic as well as killing capacity. T lymphocytes can produce lymphokine and B cell antibodies, but these are largely *in vitro* phenomena. The significant implications for the infant of these subtle differences is unclear. It is important to note that a great many basic questions have not been resolved with regard to the impact of the immunological cells on the infant's immune response: Do the cells survive in the gastrointestinal tract? Do they enter the infant's tissues? Do they modify the immune development and response? Comparative studies between breast-fed and bottle-fed infants have often yielded conflicting results.

OTHER PROTECTIVE FACTORS IN BREAST MILK

Factors with potential immunoprotective activity include lactoferrin, lysozyme, antiviral factors, lipases, oligosaccharides and gangliosides. Lactoferrin is synthesized by neutrophils and epithelial cells and is present in secretions at mucosal surfaces. Lactoferrin is the principal iron-binding protein of human milk. Lactoferrin has been shown to have an inhibitory effect on the growth of *E. coli* and *C. albicans*. This inhibitory effect is reversed by the addition of iron and, presumably, is the result of depriving organisms of iron. Lactoferrin also has a direct but bactericidal effect on some strains of bacteria, including streptococci, cholera, *Pseudomonas aeruginosa* and *C. albicans*. The presence of lactoferrin in milk is one of the several factors that alters the gastrointestinal flora of breast-fed infants, compared with bottle-fed infants.

Lysozyme

Although this has been clearly demonstrated in human milk, its role is not well understood. Its concentration in milk decreases at 1 month and, curiously, rises again at 6 months. The high levels persist in the second year of lactation.

Oligosaccharides

Recent research suggests that oligosaccharides in human milk can mimic receptors on mucosal surface epithelial cells for pathogenic invasive bacteria. It would appear that these oligosaccharides have an important role in interfering with the adhesion of bacteria to the epithelial surface. Such inhibition may interfere with colonization and provide a potential mechanism for how breast-feeding may decrease the incidence of otitis media.

Gangliosides

These are glycosphingolipids that contain sialic acid and are present in fat globule membranes in milk. Gangliosides inhibit cholera enterotoxin and *E. coli*-labile enterotoxin by interfering with binding to the mucosal cell surface receptor for the toxin.

DOES BREAST-FEEDING PROTECT THE INFANT FROM INFECTION?

Although the immunoprotective factors described above would, in theory, protect the neonate against infection, definitive information on the impact on the infant is still lacking. The difficulty in comparing breast-feeding and bottle-feeding infants involves the inability to conduct a randomized controlled study with an infant and mother assigned to a feeding method. Hence, confounding variables such as socio-economic factors, maternal smoking, family history of atopic disease and other factors necessitate large, well-designed studies to answer questions of protective effect of breast-feeding on infections and allergic diseases. The general perception, however, is that there is a significant protective activity. Severity of illness is also an important variable, since breast-feeding has been associated with a decreased rate of hospitalization in the first 3 months of life.

3

Disorders with a putative immunological basis in obstetric and gynecological practice

3.1 The immunology of recurrent spontaneous miscarriage

DEFINING RECURRENT MISCARRIAGE

Historically, a woman was said to suffer from recurrent miscarriage if she had experienced three consecutive miscarriages with the same partner, and had had no more than one live birth. If this definition is used, then 1% of the population is affected.

However, in recent years, in part due to new scientific findings and in part due to patient pressure, women who have suffered only two consecutive miscarriages with the same partner, and have had no more than one live birth, are also considered recurrent miscarriers, and many clinics will investigate such women. This increases the proportion of the population labeled as recurrent miscarriers to 3–5%.

It is unusual for women to miscarry after 14 weeks of pregnancy where a fetal heart and otherwise normal progress of the pregnancy had previously been demonstrated. It is therefore prudent to evaluate a woman who has suffered such a miscarriage, even if it was her first pregnancy. Such a woman may have a weak cervix, or other investigations may yield a treatable cause.

PROGNOSIS IN RECURRENT MISCARRIAGE

A woman who has suffered a single sporadic miscarriage (15–20% of all pregnancies end in miscarriage) has an 80% chance of her next pregnancy being successful. Other than empathy and reassurance, no other investigations or treatments are usually required.

59

If, having suffered one miscarriage, the second pregnancy also miscarries, then this woman has a 70% chance of her next pregnancy being successful.

If the woman is even more unfortunate and suffers three consecutive miscarriages, she has a 60% chance of her next pregnancy being successful.

Thus, two or three consecutive miscarriages occur more frequently than chance alone would predict, suggesting that in a proportion of these women there may be an underlying cause, warranting investigation and treatment.

An underlying cause for recurrent miscarriage is found in approximately 60% of women with recurrent miscarriage. This means that in 40% no cause is found, and this can often cause major distress to women, although in fact 'normal findings' should be reassuring, and leave a woman with a high chance of success in subsequent pregnancies.

Failure to find a cause in up to 40% of cases unfortunately also indicates the limitations in our knowledge and understanding of early-pregnancy events. Although there are some well-defined autoimmune and perhaps less well-defined alloimmune causes of recurrent spontaneous miscarriage (RSM), many suspect an undefined immune mechanism as the underlying cause in most if not all of the 40% of cases in which the standard investigative protocol fails to identify a cause. Therefore, there is intense research activity in the field of recurrent miscarriage.

CAUSES OF RECURRENT MISCARRIAGE

The known causes of recurrent miscarriage may be grouped as follows:

• Immunological

• Thrombophilia-related

• Hormonal

• Infection-related

• Anatomical

• Chromosomal

• Environmental

Non-immunological causes of RSM are discussed here briefly only for completeness. The rest of the chapter is then devoted to a discussion of the auto- and alloimmune causes.

Thrombophilias

Individuals with a thrombophilia are at increased risk of thromboembolic phenomena. This increased risk is because the individual makes too much of a clot-promoting protein, or too little of a protein that promotes dissolution of clots. Pregnancy itself, even in women without a thrombophilia, increases the risk of clot formation six-fold. So, women with a thrombophilia are at significant risk of clot formation during pregnancy.

In recent years, research has shown that thrombophilias, some of which are acquired while others are inherited, are a significant contributor to recurrent miscarriage. While it is tempting to suppose that thrombophilias impair pregnancy by the formation of blood clots around the early placenta, in reality the story is more complex. There is evidence for impairment of trophoblast function or invasion, although the exact mechanisms have yet to be elucidated. The good news is that once identified, there are effective therapeutic interventions for these disorders.

The primary antiphospholipid syndrome

This is an example of an acquired thrombophilia, the most important markers of which are the *lupus anticoagulant* and *anticardiolipin antibodies*. It is estimated that the primary antiphospolipid syndrome (PAPS) can be diagnosed in about 15% of women with recurrent miscarriage. Left untreated, women suffer a miscarriage rate of up to 90%. Earlier studies showed that treatment with a combination of low-dose aspirin and low-molecular-weight heparin gave a 70% chance of successful pregnancy, while aspirin on its own gave a 40% chance of success. Intriguingly, some recent reports have suggested that aspirin on its own can in effect achieve the high results achieved by the combination with heparin!

Factor V Leiden mutation

This is an example of an inherited thrombophilia which, in the absence of treatment, is associated with recurrent miscarriage. Factor V Leiden is carried by 5% of Caucasians, but is rarely found among black people. Again, the current approach is to treat carriers of this mutation with a combination of heparin and low-dose aspirin.

Other thrombophilias

These include protein C deficiency, protein S deficiency, antithrombin III deficiency, G20210A prothrombin gene mutation, hyperhomocysteinemia, etc. These disorders are in fact rare, and because of the small numbers no conclusive studies have been conducted to prove that they cause recurrent miscarriage. However, the pragmatic approach is to assume that if they are the only finding in a woman presenting with recurrent miscarriage, they may well be contributory. Treatment is similarly with heparin and aspirin, and if this is not given to 'cure' recurrent miscarriage, it will at least protect the woman against blood clot formation!

Hormonal causes of recurrent miscarriage

Polycystic ovaries

An ultrasound finding of polycystic ovaries (PCO) is common in the general female population: 22–25% of women will be found to have slightly enlarged ovaries with small cysts arranged around the edge rather like a necklace. PCO may be entirely without symptoms, but can also be a cause of long and/or irregular menstrual cycles, infertility, acne, difficulty with keeping weight down and hirsutism. When PCO are associated with symptoms or signs, the condition is then referred to as the polycystic ovarian syndrome or disease (PCOS or PCOD). Hormonal abnormalities associated with PCOS include increased production of luteinizing hormone (LH) and testosterone.

A link has been suggested between PCO and recurrent miscarriage because most studies have shown that PCO are over-represented in women with RSM, reports ranging from 40 to 80%. Although it is thought that high levels of LH may interfere with the normal maturation of eggs in the woman, and in this way predispose to miscarriage, research has shown that high levels of LH are not a cause of miscarriage. Thus, LH and/or PCO may simply be markers of another underlying cause. Various avenues of research are currently ongoing to elucidate the possible mechanism(s) that may be involved in recurrent miscarriage in women with PCO.

Progesterone

Progesterone is undoubtedly a key hormone in pregnancy maintenance, since the administration of drugs that abolish its activity, or removal before 6–7 weeks' gestation of the corpus luteum, which produces most of the progesterone in early pregnancy, results in miscarriage. Progesterone appears to have many roles in pregnancy, including rendering the endometrium more receptive to the early embryo, and inducing quiescence in the uterus. It is also thought to alter decidual cytokine balance in a way that tends to promote pregnancy (see section below on the immunological causes of RSM). It should not be surprising therefore that it has been suggested that low levels of progesterone may be a cause of miscarriage, sporadic or recurrent. Linked to this has been the idea of 'corpus luteum deficiency' whose diagnosis can only be made, not always reliably, by taking and carefully examining a biopsy from the lining of the womb in the second half of the menstrual cycle. For many years women were given progesterone supplements as a treatment for recurrent miscarriage, but the practice was largely abandoned when a meta-analysis showed lack of efficacy for the treatment.

Current views are that low levels of progesterone hormone reflect a pregnancy that is failing, rather than being a cause of the pregnancy failure. However, these views are being challenged again. Many have criticized the meta-analysis that showed a lack of benefit from progesterone supplementation because of the poor quality of studies included. Others have pointed to recent research that has shown very clearly that progesterone supplementation prevents late miscarriage and preterm birth in women at risk. They have argued that some cases of late miscarriage and preterm birth represent a spectrum condition that starts in the first trimester of pregnancy, and progesterone supplementation may therefore benefit a select group of women, although nobody knows how that group of women is to be identified.

This area is therefore ripe for further research. Some women, based on previous experience, are convinced that progesterone prevents recurrent miscarriage. Provided that they understand the small risks, the pragmatic approach is to allow them to use progesterone supplements. It should be remembered that progesterone support is widely used in *in vitro* fertilization (IVF) treatment cycles, where it is essential and safe, although this does not provide evidence for efficacy in RSM.

Other hormones

Poorly controlled diabetes mellitus or untreated over- and underactive thyroid gland can probably cause miscarriage. However, it would be highly unlikely that a woman with one of these diseases would present for the first time with a history of recurrent miscarriage, but be otherwise well.

Infection as a cause of recurrent miscarriage

While an acute infection causing high fever and general malaise may cause a sporadic miscarriage, chronic infection of the genital tract is rare, and therefore infection is not considered a common cause of recurrent miscarriage.

However, recent research has shown that *bacterial vaginosis* (BV) is strongly linked to a significant risk of late miscarriage (14–24 weeks) and preterm birth. BV is not considered an infection, but is a change in the normal bacterial flora in the vagina, when the healthy bacteria that are normally resident there are replaced by others that then cause a yellowish, 'fishy' smelling discharge. Although the organisms that cause BV are known, it is not known why some women get BV, and it is a condition that comes and goes. It can be treated successfully with antibiotics, but often recurs.

Earlier research suggested that antibiotic treatment of BV did not reduce the risk of late miscarriage and preterm birth, but recent and rigorous research published in

The Lancet in 2003 showed that early treatment of BV reduces both late miscarriage and preterm birth.

Anatomical causes of recurrent miscarriage

It has for a long time been debated whether congenital abnormalities of the uterus cause recurrent miscarriage. There is no doubt that women with a so-called *double uterus*, or *uterine septum*, often have successful pregnancies, but when it is the only abnormality found in a woman with RSM, it leaves doubt as to its potential role in the RSM. Other abnormalities that occur later in life, such as *polyps* and *fibroids*, may also be linked to RSM, but conclusive proof remains elusive.

Many doctors are now offering excision of a septum in a woman with RSM, especially if no other abnormality is found to account for the RSM. Submucous fibroid(s) are readily removed with hysteroscopic resection, without any negative sequelae in expert hands, and so it is prudent that any such fibroids be removed. However, fibroids in other parts of the uterus (intramural, subserous) are unlikely to cause miscarriage, and any decision for surgery must be weighed against the potential risks from surgery such as the formation of adhesions and infertility.

Cervical weakness

Previously referred to as cervical incompetence, this condition causes late miscarriages (14–24 weeks' gestation). Diagnosis is notoriously difficult, and is commonly based on a history of late miscarriages which are often painless and associated with minimal bleeding. Cervical weakness may be congenital, but the majority are acquired following trauma to the cervix such as with mechanical dilatation during repeated late-pregnancy termination, or extensive biopsy of the cervix for abnormal smears. It is likely that cervical weakness is overdiagnosed, as there is no reliable method of diagnosing the condition. Treatment involves the insertion of a stitch around the cervix, usually performed at 12–14 weeks' gestation.

Chromosome abnormalities

Approximately 60–70% of sporadic (one-off) miscarriages are caused by a chromosomal abnormality of the fetus. Errors in the transmission and division of the chromosomes can occur and lead to the fetus having either too few or too many chromosomes, which is often incompatible with life, and the pregnancy miscarries. These chromosome errors occur randomly, and in rare instances may cause recurrent miscarriage. Most research shows that the likelihood of RSM caused by chromosome abnormalities in the fetus is related to the age of the mother, and increases from 19% at ages under 35 years to 47% in women over 35 years.

In approximately 5–7% of couples with RSM, one or the other partner (more commonly the woman) possesses abnormal chromosomes which they repeatedly pass on to the fetus. The abnormality is usually not in the number of chromosomes, but in the way in which they are arranged. The commonest such rearrangement is called a *balanced translocation* (an 'inversion' is another example, but very rare). Obviously there is currently no cure for the chromosomal abnormality in the parent, but when such a parental chromosomal abnormality is identified, referral to a clinical geneticist is offered. S/he will be best placed to advise on the future prospects, and may also advise on the need for prenatal tests to detect the abnormality in any future pregnancy, as some abnormalities may be compatible with the birth of a live but incapacitated baby. The chances of a successful pregnancy in the future will depend on the specific type of chromosomal abnormality.

It should also be appreciated that current tests examine the chromosomes, but not the individual genes, of parents or fetuses. Thus, standard techniques do not pick up single-gene mutations, which may nevertheless contribute to repeated miscarriage. The future is bright – with the rapid development of DNA technology, it is likely to be possible to detect *genetic causes* for recurrent miscarriage.

Environmental causes of recurrent miscarriage

It is reasonable to suppose that any toxic substance that a woman consumes may cause miscarriage.

Heavy smoking A consumption of > 15 cigarettes/day increases the risk of miscarriage in a dose-dependent manner.

Alcohol Heavy alcohol consumption is well known to cause the 'fetal alcohol syndrome', but it is now generally believed that lower levels of alcohol consumption may also increase the risk of miscarriage, again in a dose-dependent manner.

Stress This is generally thought to increase the risk of miscarriage, but the term 'stress' can mean all sorts of things, and women have successful pregnancies in conditions which, on the face of it, should be highly stressful, such as war zones! Nevertheless, it is prudent to avoid stress whenever possible.

IMMUNOLOGICAL CAUSES OF RECURRENT MISCARRIAGE

Is an intact immune system crucial for successful pregnancy?

Whether an intact immune system is crucial for successful pregnancy is pertinent to the issue of the possible role of the immune system in RSM. Doubly homozygous scid/beige mice (scid, severe combined immunodeficiency), which lack all B cell and T cell function, and most natural killer (NK) cell activity, can reproduce successfully in the absence of infection. Mice homozygous for defective β_2-microglobulin genes, and hence incapable of classical major histocompatibility complex (MHC) class I cell-surface expression, can nevertheless develop normally *in utero*, suggesting that allo-recognition is not important in pregnancy. In humans, it has long been recognized that women with congenital or adult-onset agammaglobulinemia can have successful pregnancies. Thus, it would seem that an intact maternal immune system is not essential for successful reproduction. However, it is well established that fertility and pregnancy success are better when the parents are genetically dissimilar – the concept of hybrid vigor. Furthermore, it is clear that there are circumstances in which the immune system can be detrimental, and others in which it can be beneficial. The obvious examples of harmful effects are seen in certain types of autoimmune disease such as systemic lupus erythematosus (SLE), or in those with the antiphospholipid syndrome (APS), where early pregnancy loss is common, and those pregnancies that proceed to viability often develop complications. A further instructive example are the women with the rare p phenotype in the erythrocyte antigenic system: they make anti-PP_1P^k antibodies which cross the placenta and may be responsible for the more than 50% early pregnancy loss.

Cytokines and the Th1/Th2 cytokine balance and RSM

T lymphocytes can be classified as helper Th1 cells, which synthesize interleukin (IL)-2, interferon (IFN)-γ and tumour necrosis factor (TNF)β, and induce cellular immunity; or helper Th2 cells, which synthesize IL-4, IL-5, IL-6, IL-10 and IL-13, and induce antibody production. In what is now regarded a landmark paper, the late Thomas Wegmann and his colleagues reported in 1993 that, at least in mice and murine models, normal pregnancy is associated with the dominance of cytokines of the Th2 variety, whereas pregnancy failure was associated with Th1-type responses. Additional evidence in support of this hypothesis has since emerged from further murine studies as well as research in humans. Elevated maternal serum levels of TNFβ and/or IL-2 receptor have been reported in patients with spontaneous abortion, and unexplained RSM. Thus, the concept that first-trimester normal pregnancy is a Th2 phenomenon, whereas pregnancy failure is a Th1 phenomenon, has dominated thinking since the initial publication by Wegmann and his colleagues.

However, these concepts of the Th1/Th2 paradigm have not been translated into effective therapeutic interventions in humans. Some have looked at the example of the highly successful use of anti-TNFα (infliximab, monoclonal antibody treatment) therapy in rheumatoid arthritis, but as yet there are no reports of equivalent efficacy in the treatment of RSM. This is an expensive treatment whose potential side-effects require significant caution, and, given the uncertainties, render such attempts at therapy dangerous.

The dogma of Th2 predominance in normal pregnancy has been challenged in recent years. Of particular relevance in this regard are the two cytokines IL-12 and IL-18. At high doses, IL-12 is a Th1 cytokine that enhances the cytotoxicity of both NK and T cells and induces a high IFN-γ secretion. Yet IL-12 is expressed in the human uterus, and at least in mice appears to be required for successful implantation, since its mutation causes vascular abnormalities at the uteroplacental interface. IL-18 alone is a Th2-promoting cytokine, with positive effects on local vascular transformation by the stimulation of the production of angiopoietin 2. But IL-18 can also behave as a Th1-like cytokine, and was initially characterized as a co-stimulator factor for the induction of IL-12-mediated IFN-γ production by Th1 cells and the hyperactivation of NK cells. In recent murine studies, IFN-γ, long regarded as a major Th1 cytokine with detrimental effects in pregnancy, now appears to be a key mediator regulating gene expression in vascular and decidual tissues.

It therefore seems that the Th1/Th2 paradigm is no longer sustainable as previously understood, and it is more likely that different cytokine groups interact in a stage-specific manner to effect successful pregnancy, so that some cytokines previously thought to be of the Th1 variety and therefore detrimental to pregnancy are in fact critical for successful early pregnancy development. Moreover, given the large numbers of cytokines at the maternofetal interface, interpretation of the role of individual cytokines is likely to be fraught with errors. Clearly, a great deal of research is still required in this area, and screening the expression of multiple cytokine genes with a microarray system, and quantification of either excess or depletion of cytokines of interest by quantitative reverse transcriptase-polymerase chain reaction, offer some hope of a resolution to these major questions.

A role for the natural killer cell in RSM?

In Chapter 1, NK cells were described as being part of the innate immune system, which protect the body against viral and bacterial infection without the need for prior sensitization. In discussing the systemic inflammatory response observed in normal pregnancy (Chapter 2), it was highlighted that NK cell numbers and activity in humans have been consistently shown to be depressed. This would seem also to be consistent with the concept of normal pregnancy being a Th2 phenomenon. But in mice, uterine NK cells appear to be the main effector cells that directly or indirectly control the early steps of the implantation process: an absence of these cells or a lack of activation of these cells by T cells in the pre- and peri-implantation period results in abnormal peri-implantation and placental development. On the other hand, hyperactivation of these cells confers on them the ability to kill trophoblast cells *in vitro*, and *in vivo* may lead to abortion in a variety of animal models as well as in humans.

A strong body of recent research in women with recurrent miscarriage and/or implantation failure following IVF has suggested that there are increased numbers and activity of NK cells. These studies have been confined to either the peripheral blood or to the endometrium, and no simultaneous studies of both have been conducted to assess the correlation of the two, since what happens at the maternofetal interface may be very different from what happens in the periphery. Nonetheless, there has been consistency in showing enhanced numbers and activity at both sites, and the idea that these NK cells may play a key role in implantation failure or recurrent miscarriage is fast gaining ground, to the point where some have embarked on therapeutic strategies that aim to suppress NK cell activity using steroids. Caution, however, needs to be exercised, as there may well be stage-specific roles for NK cells (as there appears to be for cytokines), with them being essential in very early stages of decidualization, yet wreaking havoc at later stages if they occur in excess numbers or activity. A greater understanding of the role of NK cells in the decidua in normal pregnancy is urgently required before their role in pathology can be assumed, and before widespread use of interventions.

Autoimmune disease and recurrent miscarriage

Chapter 5 tackles the concept of autoimmune disease and the impact on reproduction. With regard to recurrent miscarriage, SLE is the best example of an autoimmune disease that compromises pregnancy: this includes recurrent miscarriage, poor fetal growth, intrauterine death and pregnancy complications such as pre-eclampsia. Treatment of active disease is usually with steroids, and if other markers such as the lupus anticoagulant or anticardiolipin antibody are also present, then heparin and aspirin may also be indicated as discussed above under 'Thrombophilias'. Patients with SLE and other connective-tissue disorders require specialized care and co-operation between obstetricians, rheumatologists and sometimes renal physicians.

INVESTIGATIONS FOR RECURRENT SPONTANEOUS MISCARRIAGE

Non-immunological tests

These are presented here for clarity and completeness.

Chromosome studies   Both partners are tested.

Infection screen   A vaginal swab is taken for bacterial vaginosis, and a cervical swab for *Chlamydia* (the latter has not been shown conclusively to be significant in RSM).

Full thrombophilia screen   This includes factor V Leiden mutation.

Day 3–4 blood test for a hormonal profile   This includes luteinizing hormone (LH), follicle stimulating hormone (FSH), prolactin, testosterone and sex hormone binding globulin (SHBG) and thyroid function. The day 3–4 profile allows a biochemical assessment of polycystic ovarian syndrome (LH : FSH ratio ≥ 2.5 being considered diagnostic).

Pelvic ultrasound scan   This is usually transvaginal, for anatomy of the uterus (to exclude uterine septa, submucous fibroids and congenital malformations – although many, such as bicornuate uterus, are not necessarily a cause of RSM); and to assess ovaries for PCO morphology. Although a standard real-time modern ultrasound machine will provide most of the desired information, technical innovations including three- and four-dimensional ultrasound mean that more accurate and more extensive imaging is becoming available.

Women who have suffered late miscarriage (14–24 weeks), and those in whom an ultrasound scan suggests a lesion inside the uterus such as a fibroid, polyp or septum, should be offered a *hysteroscopy* to confirm the diagnosis, and where appropriate, to deal with the lesion, e.g. resection of the septum or submucous fibroid or polypectomy.

Often other blood tests such as urea and electrolytes, thyroid function, liver function and blood glucose are performed, but they are not specific investigations for RSM, and are often uninformative. It would be unusual for a diabetic, or someone with Grave's disease, or some liver disorder, to present for the first time via a recurrent miscarriage clinic. Obviously chronic disease, such as chronic renal failure, would tend to compromise fertility and reproductive performance, but such chronic conditions are rarely a cause of repeated pregnancy failure.

IMMUNOLOGICAL TESTS FOR RECURRENT SPONTANEOUS MISCARRIAGE

Antiphospholipid antibodies

Test for these antibodies are crucial, since the APS is an established and treatable cause of recurrent miscarriage. The antiphospholipid antibodies (aPL) are a family of approximately 20 autoantibodies directed against negatively charged phospholipid-binding proteins, but only two of these are of clinical significance: the lupus anticoagulant and anticardiolipin antibodies (IgG and IgM, but not IgA subclasses). It is well recognized that there can be and often is considerable inter- and intralaboratory variation in the detection of aPL, and the laboratory assays therefore need to be performed according to international guidelines.

Antinuclear antibodies

While an antinuclear antibody (ANA) test may be part of a helpful screen for conditions such as SLE, routine testing for ANA in recurrent miscarriage is not useful. ANAs are a group of antibodies that react with various components of the cell nucleus, and are found in a substantial proportion of the population, especially the elderly, who never then appear to develop any specific immunological disease. If found in a younger population they are then more likely to be associated with the development of disease. The presence of ANA in women with recurrent miscarriage does not appear to affect pregnancy outcome.

Other autoimmune antibodies

It has been suggested that the finding of one autoantibody in a patient indicates that other autoantibodies may also be present, i.e. that some people have a predisposition to a range of autoimmune diseases (a good example being the autoimmune polyglandular syndrome, where the affected individuals possess autoantibodies which react with all steroid hormone-secreting cells). Women with this syndrome might therefore have ovarian antibodies, but while these antibodies may contribute to infertility, they have no association with recurrent miscarriage. Thyroid autoantibodies have also been thought to be linked to recurrent miscarriage, but research has shown that the prevalence of thyroid autoantibodies is similar in women with recurrent miscarriages compared with fertile controls, and pregnancy outcome is not affected by the presence of these antibodies in euthyroid women with a history of recurrent miscarriage.

Human leukocyte antigen typing

An idea that dominated thinking within reproductive immunology circles in the late 1970s and early 1980s was the concept that couples with increased human leukocyte antigen (HLA) sharing were more likely to miscarry because the woman mounted an inappropriate immune response to the conceptus. These ideas led to the introduction of immunotherapy (see 'Treatment options in recurrent miscarriage' below). However, evidence for increased parental HLA sharing, and therefore its role, in recurrent miscarriage is controversial. Approximately 50% of the published literature suggests that there is increased HLA sharing, while the other 50% suggests otherwise. Among those studies that reported increased sharing, the shared antigens varied from study to study. It is possible that in some communities with a high degree of consanguineous marriage, increased HLA sharing may be a risk factor in recurrent miscarriage, most likely because of retained deleterious recessive genes. However, it is generally accepted that in non-consanguineous marriage, increased HLA sharing is neither demonstrable nor a significant predictor of pregnancy outcome. Therefore, HLA typing is an expensive test whose benefits are dubious at best.

Cytokines and the Th1/Th2 response

The discussion above on the Th1/Th2 paradigm makes clear that there are considerable emerging data that are challenging this dogma. Although measurement of a wide range of cytokines is now automated, and therefore rapid and relatively cheap, interpretation of results is fraught with uncertainties. At present, there are no cytokine tests whose measurement can be used as a reliable tool in the management of a woman with recurrent miscarriage.

Natural killer cells

The discussion above on the potential role of NK cells in implantation failure and recurrent pregnancy loss suggests that there remains significant uncertainty. In terms of investigation, there is a need to establish whether peripheral NK cell activity correlates with uterine NK cell activity. It seems intuitively correct to suppose that it is the uterine NK cells that would be important in pregnancy outcome, yet routine testing for these, where it involves endometrial biopsies, is invasive and cumbersome. If peripheral blood NK cell activity reflects uterine NK cell activity, a simple blood test and the use of flow cytometry (see Chapter 6) would give a rapid answer.

TREATMENT OPTIONS IN RECURRENT MISCARRIAGE

Although this chapter is mainly concerned with the immunology of recurrent miscarriage, other aspects of recurrent miscarriage are included for completeness and clarity, since the picture is rarely ever purely immunological. A woman with a clearly identifiable immunological cause for her repeated miscarriages would nevertheless require psychological support, in addition to any specific immunological intervention, in any subsequent pregnancy. A given miscarriage may also have a different etiology (e.g. fetal chromosomal anomaly) even in the presence of an immunological cause.

Psychological support

Whatever the cause of recurrent miscarriage identified by investigations, it is only normal that women will be very anxious in any future pregnancy. Research has shown that psychological support reduces the risk of miscarriage. Such support may include frequent clinic visits when required, access to telephone support, and ready access to ultrasound facilities for viability confirmation. Many women find weekly ultrasound scans at specific times during what they consider their 'danger' periods to be very reassuring. There are, however, others who dread what the ultrasound might show, or even believe that ultrasound might contribute to miscarriage! Individualization is therefore the key to psychological support.

Treatment for the antiphospholipid syndrome

The current most widely used treatment involves low-dose aspirin (75 mg daily) and low-molecular-weight heparin (Fragmin® 2500 u or 5000 u daily). This treatment has been shown dramatically and significantly to improve the live-birth rate in women with recurrent miscarriage secondary to APS. Aspirin's mode of action is thought to be via its ability to reduce platelet adhesiveness, while heparin appears to have two actions: it improves trophoblast invasion and differentiation by binding to aPL, thereby resulting in successful implantation; and later in pregnancy, heparin's anticoagulant action may reduce the risk of placental thrombosis and infarction.

While earlier reports suggested that aspirin on its own was not as good as aspirin and heparin for APS, a recent report has suggested that aspirin alone may be just as good as the combined therapy. Such controversies clearly need resolution, for aspirin on its own would be vastly cheaper, have fewer side-effects, be easier to use and presumably be more acceptable to women. Available evidence suggests that the empirical use of aspirin in unselected women with recurrent miscarriage is of no benefit.

Treatment for thrombophilias

Recent evidence suggests that the factor V Leiden mutation is associated with a high risk of miscarriage, but responds to appropriate therapy. While it may be a subject of debate whether or not the other thrombophilias cause recurrent miscarriage, they increase the risk of thromboembolism in those affected. Pregnancy itself without thrombophilia increases the risk of thrombosis six-fold. Therefore it seems prudent to treat women with recurrent miscarriage in whom a thrombophilia has been identified with a combination of low-dose aspirin and low-molecular-weight heparin. Certainly, recent data would seem to suggest that such therapy benefits women with the factor V Leiden mutation and recurrent miscarriage. There is also a suggestion that a higher dose of aspirin (150 mg) might be indicated in these women. Since the risk of thromboembolism is especially high in the 6 weeks following childbirth, treatment should be continued during this time. Special precautions, such as stopping the aspirin and heparin for at least 12 h before a planned induction of labor, are taken to minimize the risk of excessive bleeding. Clotting studies should be performed prior to siting an epidural, even if more than 12 h have lapsed since the last Fragmin injection.

Treatment for a positive NK cell test

As discussed above, research evidence points to increased NK cell activity in subsets of women with recurrent miscarriage or implantation failure following successful IVF. There are no data on correlation between peripheral and uterine NK cell activity, although intuitively there is likely to be a correlation. But as with the Th1/Th2 paradigm, the picture continues to evolve. Some centers in the USA and the UK have moved a step into the therapeutic arena, and offer women steroids, presumably to 'suppress' the NK cell activity. The results of definitive trials are awaited, and until these are available, NK cell measurements and any treatments offered should be within the context of a research project.

'Immunotherapy'

The concept of immunotherapy encompasses the use of husband or pooled third-party lymphocytes to 'immunize' women with recurrent miscarriage, the use of trophoblast membrane fragments instead of lymphocytes or passive immunization with intravenous immunoglobulin (IVIG). The rationale behind lymphocyte immunization was based on increased HLA sharing, the immunization being intended to stimulate an appropriate, 'pregnancy-protective' response prior to pregnancy. Although a few centers still practice lymphocyte immunization, it is generally accepted, based on reviews and meta-analysis, that this treatment confers no benefits over placebo, is expensive and has potential serious side-effects, including transmission of infection, transfusion reaction and anaphylactic shock.

Trophoblast membrane fragment immunization was only ever practiced in a few centers, showed no benefits and died a death.

IVIG has been advocated on the basis that it might down-regulate NK cell activity (see above), eliminate immune complexes and down-regulate autoantibody production. Reports of 'success' in recurrent miscarriage, mainly emanating from the USA, have not been reproduced widely, and meta-analysis of published studies has concluded that there is no benefit over placebo from IVIG.

Treatment for cervical weakness

Where a 'weak cervix' has been diagnosed, the standard treatment is cervical cerclage at 12–14 weeks' gestation. The vast majority of cerclages are inserted via the vagina. Very occasionally, where a woman has had prior surgery to the cervix and where the cervix has become very short and is damaged and/or scarred, the cerclage may need to be inserted through the abdomen (transabdominal cervical cerclage). In the latter, a cesarean section delivery will be required, and the suture will usually be left in place until the woman completes her family. The standard suture inserted via the vagina is removed at 38 weeks and a vaginal delivery anticipated.

Management of chromosomal abnormalities

There is of course no cure for chromosomal abnormalities, but the identification of an abnormality allows for more accurate counseling and assessment of prognosis. Couples in whom a chromosomal abnormality is identified should be referred to a genetic counseling service.

Treatment when bacterial vaginosis is identified

It is well established that BV is associated with an increased risk of late miscarriage and preterm birth. Recent research has shown that early treatment of BV significantly reduces both risks, and oral clindamycin may cover a broader range of the more virulent species involved in BV than may metronidazole. There is, as yet, no definitive evidence for BV causing early miscarriage.

Other treatments available

Progesterone

Once, progesterone supplements were widely used to treat women with recurrent miscarriage. They fell into disrepute when a meta-analysis failed to show any benefit. However, a meta-analysis is only as good as the studies that are included, and many have since questioned the quality of the studies included. In addition, recent powerful research has shown that progesterone supplementation prevents late miscarriage and preterm birth in subsets of women at risk of both. Extrapolations are therefore being made to earlier pregnancy loss, and some women are being offered progesterone supplementation. However, current clinical practice dictates that progesterone supplementation should be used within the context of a clinical trial. Certainly patients should be made fully aware of current controversies and what is known about the efficacy or otherwise of such therapy.

Metformin

This is a common drug frequently used in the treatment of type II diabetes, but which in recent years has also been used in women who have insulin resistance as part of PCOS. It is an attractive therapeutic option because of simplicity of administration, hypoglycemia is rare and weight loss is promoted. There is an increasing volume of research supporting the use of metformin in a wide range of gynecological conditions including recurrent miscarriage, where some (but not all) observational studies suggest that metformin diminishes the risk of miscarriage. Although metformin crosses the placenta, as yet there has not been any evidence of teratogenicity. However, routine metformin use in the treatment of recurrent miscarriage awaits formal evaluation in prospective randomized trials.

When investigations fail to identify a cause

Some couples are disappointed when investigations fail to identify a cause of their recurrent miscarriages. In fact, not finding a cause should be seen as a very positive outcome, because then the chance of a subsequent successful pregnancy is very high. Where a couple have only had two consecutive miscarriages, when no cause is found they have at least a 70% chance of having a successful pregnancy. While the figure is slightly lower where there have been three consecutive miscarriages, nevertheless the chances of a successful pregnancy remain higher than those of further miscarriage. Psychological support is an important therapeutic strategy in these circumstances.

Alternative/complementary therapies

To date, no complementary treatment for recurrent miscarriage has been subjected to formal evaluation using standard research methodology. However, some couples will seek such treatment. While it is difficult to envisage how treatments such as aromatherapy and reflexology could cure recurrent miscarriage, nevertheless they are unlikely to cause any harm, and are certainly relaxing and soothing for women who are otherwise fraught with anxiety, stress and tension. Some investigations within the alternative therapy field often identify trace mineral deficiencies using hair, and attribute miscarriages to these deficiencies (usually deficiencies of zinc, magnesium or selenium). The treatment usually suggested involves dietary supplementation. It seems unlikely that a packet of multivitamin supplements purchased from a local pharmacy, and taken at recommended doses, could be harmful, and therefore it would seem unnecessary to discourage this approach, provided that couples appreciate the limitations of the therapy offered.

General measures

While there may be no hard scientific evidence for some of the general measures advocated, they appeal to common sense. Couples undergoing investigation and treatment for recurrent miscarriage may therefore be given the following advice:

(1) A healthy, balanced diet;

(2) Avoidance of excess caffeine, alcohol and recreational drugs;

(3) Cessation of smoking;

(4) Avoidance of stress (probably easier said than done);

(5) Regular exercise;

(6) During early pregnancy, avoidance of sexual intercourse: there is a link between sexual activity and BV, and sexual activity alters vaginal flora, even if only transiently.

SUMMARY AND OVERVIEW OF THE IMMUNOLOGY OF RECURRENT MISCARRIAGE

Knowledge and understanding of early pregnancy events remains remarkably rudimentary, although considerable progress has been made over the past decade or so. This explains why in up to 40% of couples a cause for recurrent miscarriage cannot be identified. It is therefore vital that research continues to be an integral part of the management of couples with recurrent miscarriage. New ideas on causation and treatment will continually evolve, and some novel investigations and treatments will generate fierce controversy and intense debate, but sometimes progress comes out of such situations. Couples with recurrent miscarriage, as with those with infertility, are often desperate and vulnerable, and must be protected against unproven tests and treatments. Yet without research and treatment trials no progress can be made. The key is to make clear distinctions between research and standard therapy, and to ensure that patients also can distinguish the two.

3.2 The immunology of pre-eclampsia

INTRODUCTION

Pre-eclampsia (PE) is a major contributor to maternal and perinatal mortality and morbidity. It complicates 5% of first pregnancies, but also occurs in multiparous women. One-third of the babies are premature, and 20–30% are small for gestational age. PE is associated with a 3–10-fold increase in perinatal mortality. Serious maternal morbidity may result, and maternal mortality from this condition is common in the developing world. Finally, women who develop PE are at increased risk of developing hypertension in later life, with the attendant morbidity and mortality from cardiovascular disease. While it is popularly regarded as an 'immunological disease' among obstetricians and others, in reality PE remains the quintessential disease of theories.

Successful pregnancy is critically dependent upon profound hemodynamic changes that reflect the maternal cardiovascular adaptation to the needs of both the mother and the fetus. Such changes include marked peripheral vasodilatation accompanied by increases in blood volume, cardiac output, heart rate and decreased systemic arterial blood pressure. In healthy pregnancy, blood pressure decreases in mid-gestation, and skin perfusion increases. PE represents a failure of these adaptive responses, but the underlying mechanisms are poorly understood. The placenta, or more specifically trophoblastic tissue, is the '*sine qua non*' of PE. At present, there are two phenomena that are universally accepted as characteristic of the disease:

(1) Defective/impaired trophoblastic invasion – the single consistent histopathological feature of the syndrome (Figure 3.1);

(2) Generalized endothelial cell dysfunction – a hallmark of the disease process.

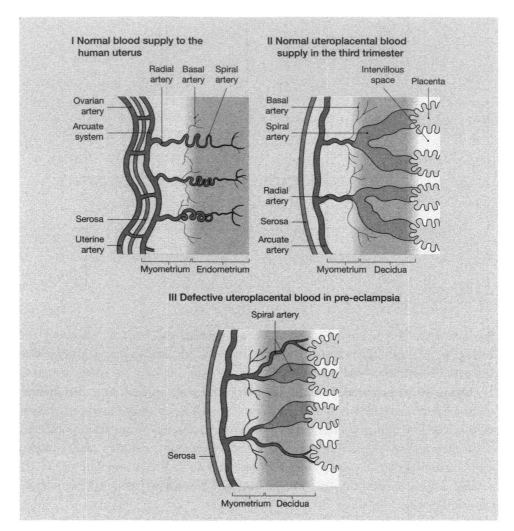

Figure 3.1 Blood supply to the uterus and normal and abnormal uteroplacental circulation. I. Anatomy of the normal blood supply to the human uterus. Note the coiled nature of the spiral artery in the non-pregnant state. II. Normal uteroplacental blood supply in the third trimester: cytotrophoblastic cells (invasive or endovascular trophoblast) have migrated into the decidual and myometrial segments of the spiral arteries which they have converted into uteroplacental arteries – this process takes place in the first and second trimester; the morphological changes which are adaptations to pregnancy are referred to as 'physiological changes'. The endovascular trophoblast penetrates the vessel wall through the endothelial lining and disrupts the intima, internal elastic lamina and much of the muscular media, and deposits a fibrinoid material. The result is a dilated, flaccid uteroplacental vasculature unresponsive to vasomotor influences, associated with a significant drop in peripheral resistance and thus creating a low pressure zone to accommodate the 10-fold increase in blood supply to the fetoplacental unit. III. Defective physiological changes seen in PE (and also in pregnancies complicated by intrauterine growth restriction without PE, and in some diabetic pregnancies). Some spiral arteries are totally devoid of physiological changes throughout their course while others have physiological changes restricted to the decidual segments. Since defective physiological changes are a consistent histopathological feature of PE, it is reasonable to assume that they are central to the pathophysiology

The clinical manifestations are simple enough to explain: the hypertension arises from generalized vasoconstriction, the proteinuria is due to glomerular damage and the edema is a consequence of increased vascular permeability. But why trophoblastic invasion should be defective remains a great enigma, and will probably remain so until the regulation of normal trophoblastic invasion is better understood. The mechanisms by which endothelial cell dysfunction is mediated also remain open to conjecture and speculation. A number of key observations would persuade one to consider that significant immunological aberrations could explain this condition:

(1) The historical 'primiparity only' concept of PE;

(2) The newer notion of a 'primipaternity-related disease';

(3) The impact of birth interval on risk of PE;

(4) The concept of seminal 'priming' for protection against PE;

(5) A potential role for human leukocyte antigen (HLA)-DR (and HLA-G) in PE.

While the basis of impaired or defective trophoblastic invasion remains an enigma, data from a great deal of recent research point to a number of mechanisms by which the widespread endothelial cell dysfunction seen in PE may occur. The current key concepts include the following:

(1) Oxidative stress induced by the placental hypoxia consequent from impaired trophoblastic invasion;

(2) The concept of PE as an exaggeration of the inflammatory response seen in normal pregnancy;

(3) Cytokine imbalance, with helper Th1 predominance, which might mediate some of the essential features of the syndrome;

(4) A potential role for dyslipidemia.

It is appealing to consider that most, if not all, of these phenomena are in fact interlinked, and that there may be a unifying hypothesis that goes a long way to explaining the pathophysiology of PE. All the issues above are discussed in this chapter, and an attempt made to draw up such a unifying model of PE.

PRIMIPARITY VERSUS PRIMIPATERNITY VERSUS BIRTH-INTERVAL HYPOTHESIS IN PRE-ECLAMPSIA

Historically, PE has been considered a disease of the first pregnancy. This concept was attractive from an immunological point of view, supporting the notion of a novel antigenic challenge that gave rise to PE in first pregnancies, with tolerance being developed for subsequent pregnancies. It remains a truism that nulliparity greatly increases a woman's risk of developing PE when compared with multiparity, but much research has now shown that, although at lower risk, it is the multiparous woman who often develops severe disease and, relative to her risk of PE, has a higher risk of severe morbidity and mortality. The concept of 'primiparity' has given way to the 'primipaternity' hypothesis which stipulates an increased risk of PE upon change of partner. Thus, a woman who has PE in her first pregnancy is more likely to have PE again, or indeed for the first time, in a second pregnancy if this is by a new partner. The hypothesis would explain this risk on the basis of new antigenic challenge. More recent research from Latin America and the Scandinavian countries, based largely on birth registries, has produced evidence for the 'birth-interval hypothesis', which stipulates an increased risk of PE with increasing birth interval. A birth interval of 10 years or more was reportedly associated with an increased risk of PE, and a change of paternity for the second pregnancy was associated with a reduced risk of PE after controlling for the birth interval. Thus, this hypothesis directly challenged the primipaternity hypothesis, and argued that the apparent increase in PE risk associated with a new partner was due to failure to control for birth interval.

However, there are problems with the birth-interval hypothesis. Primipaternity may in fact be a significant but unrecognized underlying factor, since data derived from registries cannot prove paternity, and it is well known that in Western societies as many as 30% of children born in apparently stable couples are not the offspring of the putative husband. The very fact of a prolonged birth interval may suggest different paternity, or may point to a selected population of women who could have had several miscarriages before the successful index pregnancy – such women are known to have an increased risk of adverse pregnancy outcome in subsequent ongoing pregnancies. Paradoxically, a group of researchers have reported that among women without PE in their first pregnancy, changing partners increased their risk of PE by as much as 30% in the subsequent pregnancy compared with those who did not change partner, while among those women with PE in their first pregnancy, changing partners reduced PE by as much as 30% in the subsequent pregnancy! Thus, the controversy of the primipaternity versus birth-interval hypotheses can only be resolved by large-scale prospective studies where paternity can be proven – a well-nigh impossible task!

SEMINAL 'PRIMING': A MECHANISM FOR PROTECTION AGAINST PRE-ECLAMPSIA?

It has been reported in recent years that the incidence of PE decreases as the duration of sexual cohabitation before conception increases. It has been hypothesized that partner-specific seminal 'priming' somehow confers protection against PE. This concept is consistent with observations that a woman is at higher risk of developing PE after insemination with donor sperm compared with partner sperm. Egg donation also increases the risk of PE, and embryo donation even more dramatically – in this instance the entire fetal genome is allogeneic.

If it is accepted that the average duration of sexual cohabitation before conception in a human couple is 7–8 months (these data come from demographers and the World Health Organization (WHO)) with sexual intercourse occurring twice a week, and given the life expectancy of sperm in the female genital tract of 3–4 days, the human female is constantly exposed to seminal and sperm antigens for 7–8 months before conception. From a simplistic immunological viewpoint, it could be supposed that such repeated or constant exposure to seminal and sperm antigens might sensitize the female genital mucosal immune system, and thereby interfere with fertility, implantation and subsequent development of a pregnancy. Such deleterious sensitization clearly does not occur. Indeed, there is increasing evidence that the converse is in fact the case – that repeated exposure activates maternal immune responses in a manner that positively supports pregnancy success, while lack of adequate exposure might compromise a pregnancy. It appears that vaginal intercourse may not be the only manner in which semen can improve reproductive outcome, since it has been reported that oral sex is also associated with a diminished incidence of PE, provided that semen contains normal levels of HLA.

What is the mechanism by which seminal and/or sperm antigens might elicit the apparently protective immune responses? Other than the observations described above, there are precious few data from humans because of the obvious difficulties of designing the kind of experiment that might provide the answers. Most available data therefore come from the rodent model, in which it is now well documented that semen triggers an influx of antigen-presenting cells into the female reproductive tract which process and present paternal ejaculate antigens to elicit activation of lymphocytes in the adaptive immune compartment. Activated T lymphocytes with a paternal antigen-specific hyporesponsiveness have been demonstrated in lymph nodes draining the uterus. Evidence suggests that transforming growth factor-β (TGFβ), a cytokine present in abundance in seminal plasma, initiates this inflammatory response by stimulating the synthesis of pro-inflammatory cytokines and chemokines in uterine tissues. The same cytokine, which is known to possess potent immune-deviating effects, may be crucial in skewing the immune response against a Th1 bias. Prior exposure to semen in the context of TGFβ has been shown to be associated with enhanced fetal–placental development late in gestation. There is no rodent model of PE, and placentation in rodents is significantly different from that in humans, but the experimental findings in rodents and the clinical observations would tend to suggest that extrapolation from the rodent to the human is not altogether unreasonable.

In summary, the clinical observation of increased risk of PE in association with donor insemination and egg and embryo donation, the apparent decrease in risk of PE with longer duration of sexual cohabitation prior to conception and the evidence from the rodent model all support the hypothesis that seminal exposure induces a partner-specific immune response which is protective towards the fetoplacental unit, including reducing the risk of developing PE.

HUMAN LEUKOCYTE ANTIGEN AND PRE-ECLAMPSIA

HLA-DR

HLA-DR antigens play a central role in self- and non-self-recognition, and in rejection reactions. It has been reported that women who develop PE and their partners show a statistically significant increase in HLA-DR homozygosity and reduced antigenic variety compared with controls, suggesting further that PE is a partner-specific disease.

HLA-G

Although this non-polymorphic MHC molecule has received a great deal of attention from the point of view of reproductive immunology, its exact role or function remains an enigma. Pieces of data accumulate all the time. With regard to PE, recent research suggests that expression of HLA-G protein is reduced in term pre-eclamptic placentas compared with placentas from normotensive pregnancies, but the significance of this with regard to the pathophysiology of PE remains obscure. Interesting observations include the finding that the soluble HLA-G1 isoform down-regulates both CD8+ and CD4+ T cell reactivity, and also down-regulates endothelial cell proliferation and migration. HLA-G also modulates innate immunity by binding to several NK and/or decidual receptors, inducing particular cytokine secretion. Given the discussion below on pathophysiological mechanisms of PE, it seems probable that HLA-G may play an important role in PE, although the processes involved are far from being elucidated.

PATHOPHYSIOLOGICAL MECHANISMS IN PRE-ECLAMPSIA

Oxidative stress in PE

There is now ample evidence for oxidative stress in PE. Oxidative stress is a biochemical imbalance which arises either from excessive generation of free radicals and/or inadequate endogenous antioxidant capacity. Free radicals are species capable of independent existence that contain free electrons, rendering them highly reactive. Examples include superoxide (O_2) and hydroxyl (OH) radicals, which create the most havoc biologically, and are termed reactive oxygen species (ROS). They are either oxygen-containing free radicals (containing an unpaired and highly reactive electron) or non-radicals, which lack the spare electron (e.g. hydrogen peroxide, H_2O_2). Although the unopposed radical species have only a transient existence, they are a dangerous entity. ROS attempt to establish a steady state by extracting an electron from an adjacent non-radical molecule to form a stable pair in its outer orbit. This converts the non-radical into a radical, often precipitating a chain reaction, with the spare electron being passed from molecule to molecule. Hydrogen atoms are the prime target for radicals as they have a single available electron, but removal of this electron disrupts chemical bonds and threatens molecular structure. There are numerous sources of free radicals, including enzymatic and mitochondrial sources. The latter are probably one of the most important sources of superoxide since they continually 'leak' spare electrons from the electron transport chain; for example, the aging process is associated with damage to mitochondrial proteins and DNA, rendering more electrons available for donation to oxygen and the formation of superoxide.

A wide range of antioxidants has evolved to counteract the potential damage that would otherwise be caused by ROS. The commonest examples of these antioxidants include ascorbic acid (vitamin C) and α-tocopherol (vitamin E). These act by being able to donate an electron to ROS, so preventing ROS-induced cell damage, while themselves being converted to less harmful end-products (e.g. ascorbate donates an electron and is itself converted to the less harmful ascorbyl, which is subsequently metabolized to harmless end-products). There are of course a wide range of other compounds that act as antioxidants, including enzymes, but a discussion of these is beyond the scope of this chapter.

Evidence for oxidative stress in PE is provided by the raised levels of markers of lipid peroxidation (raised titers of antibodies to oxidized low-density lipoprotein (LDL); high levels of malondialdehyde; increased plasma concentrations of iso-prostane, etc). Research indicates that there are several potential sources of ROS in PE including the placenta, leukocytes (leukcocyte activation occurs in normal pregnancy and is exaggerated in PE, and such activation is invariably associated with ROS generation) and the endothelium (endothelial cells synthesize superoxide via the reduced nicotinamide–adenine dinucleotide phosphate (NADPH) oxidase pathway in both physiological and pathological situations).

Oxidative stress could account for most of the clinical features of PE. ROS can cause direct cell damage by altering DNA bases, by breaking DNA strands, by disrupting hydrogen bonds and by destabilizing membrane structure. ROS also activate apoptotic and necrotic pathways by increasing cell calcium concentration. The increased apoptosis generates cellular particles which themselves further increase leukocyte and endothelial cell activation and damage. ROS attack on polyunsaturated lipids in membranes of cells and cell organelles results in the production of lipid peroxides, which are thought to mediate most of the damage in PE. Lipid peroxides interact directly with endothelial cells to cause activation and increased permeability, and induce expression of several inflammatory cytokines and cell adhesion molecules. Leukocyte activation and adhesion then follow, together with platelet activation and edema. The central role of lipid peroxides is demonstrated by the fact that there is a five-fold increase in their plasma concentration in PE, compared with normotensive controls.

The significance of oxidative stress in the pathophysiology of PE has been underlined by the successful prevention of PE using antioxidants supplementation. In a major randomized controlled trial published in *The Lancet* in 1999, women at risk of developing PE and given 1000 mg vitamin C and 400 iu vitamin E showed a highly significant reduction in the incidence of PE compared with those given placebo.

PE as an exaggerated inflammatory response

It is now generally recognized that systemic inflammation is a feature of normal pregnancy, and the nature of this inflammatory response is described in Chapter 2. The same research group that crystallized this concept in the late 1990s has now suggested that PE is quite simply an exaggeration of the normal inflammatory response of pregnancy. Their hypothesis suggests that PE develops when the systemic inflammatory process, common to all women in the second half of pregnancy, becomes so exaggerated that it causes one or other maternal system to decompensate.

This attractive hypothesis requires an appreciation of the nature of the systemic inflammatory response – a generalized activation of the innate immune system which includes monocytes and granulocytes, the complement system, platelets, the coagulation system and the *endothelium*. When discussing the innate immune system, immunologists do not usually include the endothelium, but in fact endothelial cells possess many of the receptors that are activated as part of the innate system response, can present antigen upon appropriate stimulation, produce a range of pro-inflammatory cytokines and can stimulate and be stimulated by inflammatory leukocytes. This then allows the central dogma of endothelial cell dysfunction being the hallmark of PE to be explained within the context of an exaggerated inflammatory response – the endothelium controls and regulates the micro-circulation via synthesis and release of potent vasoconstrictor substances such as thromboxane-A2 and endothelin-1. Since pro-inflammatory stimuli can impair endothelial-dependent relaxation, it becomes obvious how an exaggerated inflammatory response can result in decompensation and allows most, if not all, of the clinical features of the PE syndrome to be explained.

An important question is how this concept of an exaggerated inflammatory response relates to oxidative stress, dealt with in the section above, especially as many of the processes involved in the latter are an intrinsic part of the former and vice versa: oxidative stress can stimulate an inflammatory response, while an inflammatory response generates oxidative stress. There are mediators common to both processes (e.g. ROS); control processes common to both (e.g. the transcription factor NFκB is activated by hypoxia and oxidative stress, and controls many immune and inflammatory responses); and substances that demonstrate antioxidant activity (vitamins C and E) also have intrinsic anti-inflammatory activity – they will therefore counter both the oxidative stress and inflammatory activity seen in PE. When they are shown to prevent PE (see section on 'Oxidative stress' on p. 85), it is open to speculation whether they do so via their antioxidant action or via their anti-inflammatory activity. To those who seek unifying hypotheses, this is in fact a potentially attractive situation (see 'Towards a unifying hypothesis' on p. 90).

What is the stimulus for the exaggerated inflammatory response of pre-eclampsia?

For obvious reasons already dealt with above, whatever the nature of the stimulus, it must originate from the placenta. It should also be found in all pregnancies to explain the 'normal' inflammatory reaction of normal pregnancy, and for obvious reasons should be found in excessive amounts in PE. The research group who proposed the exaggerated inflammatory response hypothesis has provided experimental data that strongly suggest that syncytiotrophoblast microparticles (STBMs) may be a key stimulus. STBMs are found in the plasma of normal pregnant women, but their levels are significantly increased in PE. They can exact direct endothelial cell damage, and may also have pro-inflammatory activity. It is now also well established that in addition to the high levels of STBMs, PE is also associated with increased levels of cellular, subcellular and molecular debris, which are also found but at lower levels in normal pregnancy. This debris is now thought to result from syncytial apoptosis and necrosis, both processes occurring in normal pregnancy, but exaggerated in PE. While apoptosis is thought to play a central role in the normal turnover of cytotrophoblast and renewal of the syncytial surface of chorionic villi, it has been proposed that the hypoxia in the placenta of pre-eclamptic pregnancy accelerates this process, with consequent release of placental debris, which acts as a stimulus of the systemic inflammatory response.

While the evidence for innate immune system activation in normal pregnancy is now incontrovertible, and attractive though the hypothesis of an exaggerated inflammatory response as the basis of PE might be, many questions are left unanswered. Why, for example, should the exaggerated response be mainly confined to first pregnancies (or the first pregnancy with a new partner)? Might activation of the innate immune system not simply be an epiphenomenon, because if exaggeration of the activation were an important cause of PE, would PE not occur more frequently? It has been suggested that activation of the innate system in pregnancy helps to protect the mother against infection, yet in fact it puts the mother at risk not only of PE, but of exaggerated responses to other otherwise common infections, resulting in immunopathology (see Chapter 5).

Th1/Th2 cytokine imbalance in pre-eclampsia

In Chapter 2.1, a role for a Th2 cytokine predominance in successful pregnancy was discussed, when it was suggested that a Th1 predominance was associated with pregnancy failure in the form of miscarriage. If one considers that certain pregnancy disorders may be a continuum manifesting differently in each trimester, then it might not be all that surprising that a cytokine imbalance could also be found in PE. Thus, a profound Th1 predominance in the first trimester might result in miscarriage, but if the fetus survives, then the same imbalance might cause PE in the late second trimester and third trimester. This has indeed been reported: the levels of Th1 cytokine TNFα have been shown to be increased, as well as enhancement of IL-12 and IL-18 levels. A clear increase in Th1 versus Th2 cells has been reported, and this increase appears to predate the onset of the clinical disease. The picture becomes somewhat more complex, as it has been reported that there are in fact two types of pre-eclamptic profiles: the classical Th1-dominant pathways observed mostly in primiparous women, and a Th2-dominant profile, associated with high levels of anticardiolipin antibodies, and observed mostly in multiparous women.

However, it does seem unlikely that PE could be a purely cytokine-driven state, especially in the light of data showing the potential role of oxidative stress and exaggerated inflammatory responses. On the face of it, the Th1/Th2 paradigm creates a contradiction with the concept of a chronic inflammatory response in normal pregnancy. Th1 response would be expected to drive a chronic inflammatory response, yet normal pregnancy is a Th2 phenomenon. It has been proposed that perhaps Th1 responses in normal pregnancy are suppressed by STBMs, but that excess stimulation of monocytes overwhelms this and leads to Th1 activation in PE.

If there is apparent confusion with regard to the relative roles of Th1 activity and an exaggerated inflammatory response in PE, it is noteworthy that the Th1/Th2 paradigm has in recent years been challenged. For example, quadruple knock-out mice lacking IL-4, -5, -9 and -13 challenge the concept of Th2 predominance in pregnancy, since these mice have normal reproductive performance. Extensive microarray studies, which allow simultaneous analysis of large numbers of different cytokines, do indeed suggest that the Th1/Th2 paradigm no longer provides a universal explanation. It is more likely that pregnancy and implantation involve stage-specific cytokine profiles, and indeed there is growing evidence for a central role for IL-12/IL-18 regulation of uterine NK cell vascular remodeling in the human decidua.

A role for dyslipidemia

There is evidence of excess fat accumulation in several tissues in PE:

(1) 'Acute atherosis' is a classic pathological lesion seen in the placental bed in PE, resulting from the accumulation of lipid-laden macrophages surrounded by areas of fibrinoid necrosis in the spiral arteries (these features are similar to the atherogenesis in non-pregnant women, and men).

(2) 'Endotheliosis' is a characteristic lesion in the glomerulus which involves the accumulation of lipids within glomerular endothelial cells.

(3) Excess lipid accumulation in the liver occurs more prominently in severe cases of PE (e.g. in association with the HELLP syndrome – hemolysis, elevated liver enzymes and low platelet count).

The lipid accumulation at sites of endothelial damage would suggest that a disturbance of lipid metabolism may play a major role in the vascular injury seen in PE. It is now well recognized that plasma triglyceride concentrations are significantly higher in PE compared with normotensive pregnancy, and that high-density lipoprotein (HDL) cholesterol concentrations are lower in PE. Very significantly, both changes have been shown to occur in advance of the clinical manifestation of the syndrome. It should be appreciated that normal pregnancy is characterized by a change in lipid metabolism, with rises in plasma cholesterol and triglyceride concentrations thought to be due to increased lipolysis (stimulated by human placental lactogen) and/or decreased peripheral catabolism, and this rise may reflect the importance of these lipids as metabolic precursors to meet the demand of the growing fetus. Theoretical considerations of pathological dyslipidemia contributing to the PE syndrome are beyond the scope of this chapter. It is sufficient, therefore, to summarize current thoughts.

A factor(s) released from the placenta enhances peripheral lipolysis over and above that already seen in normal pregnancy, and is exacerbated by adiposity in women at risk. The lipolysis causes an increased flux of non-esterified fatty acids to the liver, where they are synthesized into triglycerides, with increased secretion into the circulation of triglyceride-rich lipoproteins (very-low-density lipoprotein, VLDL), as well as accumulation in the hepatocytes. The high levels of triglycerides in the peripheral circulation drive the production of an atherogenic lipoprotein profile by stimulating the excessive synthesis of small, dense, LDL-III and by lowering HDL cholesterol. The abnormal lipid profile may contribute to the PE syndrome as follows:

(1) Direct endothelial cell damage: small-density lipoproteins have been shown to cause direct damage to endothelial cells;

(2) Enhancement of placental production of pro-inflammatory mediators: activated macrophages (some of which accumulate lipids to become 'foam cells') and other inflammatory cells are activated and exacerbate the inflammation of normal pregnancy (see above);

(3) Potentiation of oxidative stress, via lipid peroxidation and the generation of free radicals.

TOWARDS A UNIFYING HYPOTHESIS

The discussions above clearly indicate links between oxidative stress, an exaggerated inflammatory response, a role of cytokines and a potential contribution from dyslipidemia in PE. It is very tempting to attempt to draw up a hypothesis that unifies all these concepts. Figure 3.2A–D is an attempt to do so. However, no hypothesis

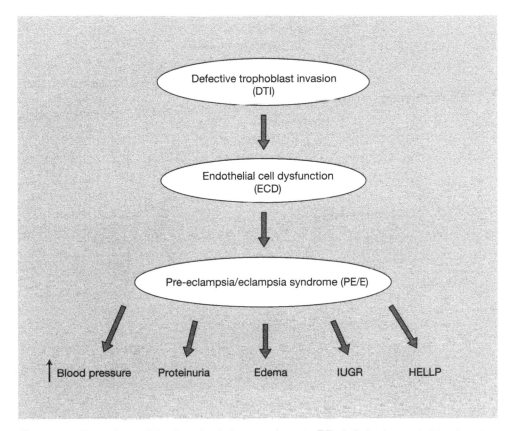

Figure 3.2 Towards a unifying hypothesis for pre-eclampsia (PE). **A.** Defective trophoblast invasion is the single consistent histopathological lesion in PE. Endothelial cell damage and dysfunction is a hallmark of the PE syndrome. The clinical features making up the PE/E syndrome are well established. Thus this figure illustrates those features of the PE/eclampsia (E) syndrome that are well-established and are not subject to speculation. IUGR, intrauterine growth restriction; HELLP, hemolysis, elevated liver enzymes and low platelet count. (*Continued*)

currently explains why trophoblast invasion is defective in the first place, and why it is largely confined to first pregnancies or a change of partner.

CONCLUDING REMARKS

It is very likely that immunological mechanisms are involved in the pathophysiology of PE. There is a wealth of research that demonstrates and implicates immunological processes, from exaggerated inflammatory responses to inappropriate cytokine activation. However, much of the data available appear to point to downstream

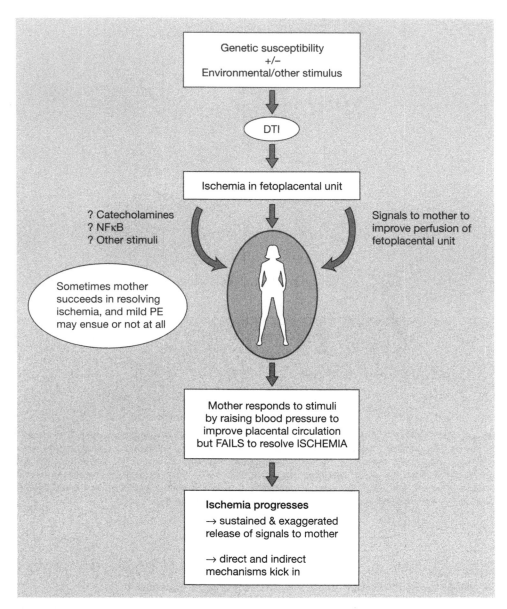

Figure 3.2 (continued) **B.** This figure builds on part A. It is not known why sometimes trophoblast invasion is defective, leading to PE, but familial predisposition suggests that genetic factors are involved, while the change of partner suggests external immunological and/or environmental influences. It is generally accepted that defective trophoblast invasion (DTI) causes ischemia within the fetoplacental unit, and it is teleologically sound to suppose that the latter sends out biological signals to the pregnant woman to resolve the ischemia. Some research has suggested that such signals might be catecholamines or NFκB but whatever they are they must result in a rise in maternal blood pressure to increase placental perfusion. When the maternal response fails to resolve the ischemia, there is presumably a sustained and exaggerated release of the biological signals, which in part will account for the sustained raised blood pressure, while the continued ischemia causes changes or responses that contribute to the PE/E syndrome. (*Continued*)

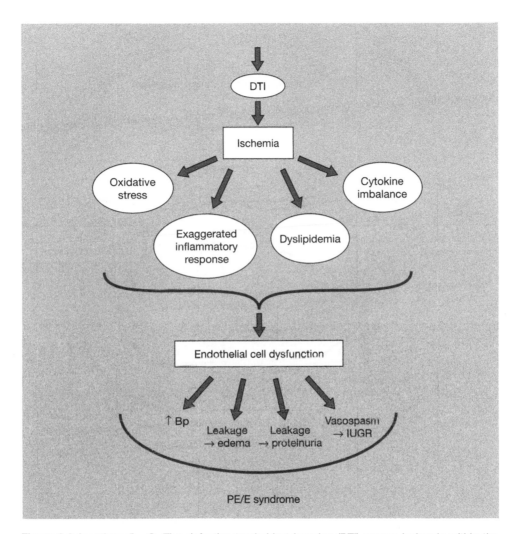

Figure 3.2 (continued)   C. The defective trophoblast invasion (DTI) causes ischemia within the fetoplacental unit. The persistent ischemia may then result in oxidative stress, an exaggeration of the normal inflammatory reaction of pregnancy, dyslipidemia and a cytokine imbalance with a Th1 predominance. These changes all contribute to the endothelial cell damage and dysfunction, the hallmark of the PE/E syndrome. Since endothelial cells play a major role in the control of blood pressure especially in the microcirculation, dysfunction contributes to the sustained raised blood pressure. Cell damage results in leaky vessels with consequent edema, and similar damage in the kidneys results is proteinuria, while vasospasm further compromises fetoplacental perfusion and the delivery of nutrients, causing intrauterine growth restriction (IUGR). (*Continued*)

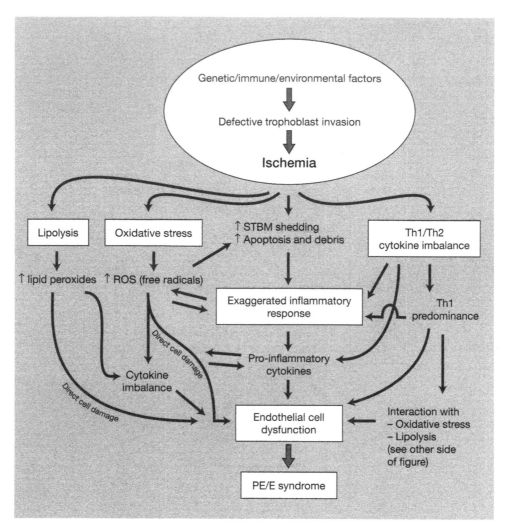

Figure 3.2 (continued)   D. This figure illustrates the potential interactions between the various key mechanisms that are thought to contribute to the PE/E syndrome, namely oxidative stress, an exaggerated inflammatory response, dyslipidemia and cytokine imbalance. Ischemia induces oxidative stress, with the resultant free radicals not only being capable of causing direct endothelial cell damage, but also promoting the exaggerated inflammatory response, increasing apoptosis and the generation of debris that contributes to the inflammatory response. Ischemia also causes increased shedding of syncytiotrophoblast microparticles (STBMs) as well as promoting apoptosis, both of which may also directly damage endothelium as well promoting the exaggerated inflammatory response, which generates pro-inflammatory cytokines which damage the endothelium. Catecholamines released as biological signals to the mother by the ischemic fetoplacental unit cause lipolysis, but other mechanisms via oxidative stress may also be implicated in the lipolysis which generates lipid peroxides, which can cause direct endothelial cell damage as well as acting via the promotion of cytokine imbalance. The cytokine imbalance in favor of the Th1 predominance may be primary or secondary, as illustrated in the figure. The contributions of the various mechanisms will presumably vary depending on the degree of ischemia, and therefore severity of the defect in trophoblast invasion. It is likely that in some situations the physiological response of the mother resolves the ischemia, and then only mild or no PE ensues

events, explaining how the disease might be mediated, but not how or why the disease occurs in the first place. The great challenge is to work out the processes that regulate normal trophoblast invasion, as this is likely to shed light on why it sometimes fails, leading to PE.

SUGGESTED FURTHER READING

Critchley H, MacLean A, Poston L, Walker J, eds. Pre-eclampsia. London: RCOG Press, 2003

3.3 Immunological infertility

INTRODUCTION

Given the central role that the immune system is thought to play in reproduction, it is reasonable to suppose that aberrant immune responses might cause infertility. In reality, immunological causes of infertility in the human female are very rare, and this section therefore largely concentrates on the male. Of the one in ten couples experiencing difficulty in conceiving, sperm antibodies (SpAbs) are regarded as one of the commonest known causes of male infertility. Prevalence rates of SpAbs in infertile men range between 6 and 11%, but SpAbs are rare in fertile couples, implying, but not proving, a role for SpAbs in infertility. Potential mechanisms of fertility impairment include diminished sperm vitality, motility and mucus penetration, and impaired sperm–egg interaction. While SpAbs can be an intractable problem, they can also be 'benign', in that natural fertility can occur in their presence. Our lack of understanding of the specific sperm antigens involved, and the functional significance of antibodies reactive with them, is a fundamental problem that has frustrated the development of SpAb testing procedures which allow the clinician to gauge precisely the relevance of SpAbs in a particular couple. Treatment procedures have accordingly been 'blunt instruments' until recent immunosuppressive therapy and, nowadays, intracytoplasmic sperm injection (ICSI) – the success of which has reduced the impetus to define the physiology of SpAbs.

IMMUNOLOGICAL INFERTILITY IN THE FEMALE

The occurrence of antiovarian autoantibodies, causing autoimmune gonaditis and hypogonadism, is often seen as a component part of the autoimmune polyglandular

97

syndrome. The latter is characterized by the presence of autoantibodies reactive with steroid hormone-secreting cells. Antiovarian antibodies can of course cause premature ovarian failure and therefore infertility. However, outside the context of autoimmune polyglandular syndrome, there is no clear evidence that ovarian antibodies cause infertility. It has been suggested that a subset of women with excessive natural killer cell activity may have successful IVF, but failure of implantation. Aberrations of the Th1/Th2 cytokine balance have also been thought to contribute to infertility, but both of these issues are linked to recurrent miscarriage, and are therefore dealt with in detail in the relevant chapter. Antisperm antibodies can also be found in women, and their possible role in female infertility is addressed below.

IMMUNOLOGICAL INFERTILITY IN THE MALE

Origin of sperm antibodies

Many sperm proteins do not arise until spermatogenesis commences at puberty, well after the development of neonatal immune tolerance. Crude sperm protein preparations are highly immunogenic in all species. So what mechanisms are normally in place to modify the immune response and prevent SpAb formation? First, there is effective separation of sperm and the immune system, starting with the occlusive Sertoli cell junctions, which effectively isolate the developing germ cells from the testicular interstitium. Less tight intercellular junctions exist within the rete testes, vas deferens ducts and epididymis. The disruption of these junctions, particularly within the epididymis, due to inflammation, trauma or a rise in hydrostatic pressure following obstruction, may result in the exposure of sperm proteins to the immune system.

However, there is considerable evidence that, under normal circumstances, some interaction occurs between sperm and the immune system within both the testes and epididymis and that immunomodulatory mechanisms act to prevent SpAb formation. Potential mechanisms for this process are ill understood, but it is clear that the presence of immunosuppressive cytokines in the testes and seminal fluid may play a role. Even less known is the environment within the epididymis. Antigen-presenting macrophages are infrequent in the normal epididymal epithelium, but prevalent in the stroma. Sperm are deficient in MHC-1 and -2 antigens required for recognition by lymphocytes. Most T lymphocytes throughout the male tract, and particularly in the epididymal epithelium, are of the suppressor/cytotoxic phenotype, but T helper cells are present in the epididymal interstitium. Whether normal resident epididymal macrophages express co-stimulatory molecules is unclear, but phagocytosis of sperm by epididymal macrophages may represent a pathway for lymphocyte activation and antibody generation. Complement-mediated destruction of sperm is thought to be minimal, as complement levels are extremely low in normal epididymal luminal fluid. Furthermore, sperm contain high levels of complement-regulatory proteins, which arise during spermatogenesis or which attach to sperm following their secretion by the epididymal epithelium.

The identification of specific biologically relevant sperm antigens has been pursued using serum from men and women with presumed immunological infertility. However, attempts to identify a universal or widely clinically relevant antigen––antibody interaction associated with infertility has, thus far, been unsuccessful. A number of candidate proteins have been identified which localize to different locations (sperm surface, head, tail components) and may arise during spermatogenesis or as a result of the incorporation of epididymal proteins. Recently, a SpAb from infertility patients was found to be directed against an epididymal glycoprotein, which shares its protein core with a CD52 lymphocyte surface molecule.

SpAbs are most commonly found after vasectomy: they occur in > 70% of men. In some of these men, these SpAbs can result in immunological infertility, despite a technically successful vasectomy reversal. The sequence of events occurring after vasectomy has been recently reviewed. Briefly, epididymal congestion is followed by minute tubal 'blow-outs' and the production of sperm granulomas, which are frequently present at the vasectomy site or within the epididymis. The latter comprise decaying sperm surrounded by macrophages and connective tissue with lymphocytes and plasma cells, and thus permit interaction between sperm proteins and the immune system. However, SpAbs can also occur in the absence of granulomas. Phagocytosis of sperm also occurs within the epididymal lumen, and changes in interaction of lymphocyte populations and in the intercellular junction normally separating sperm from the immune cells are also seen.

Other known risk factors for SpAb formation include:

(1) Any cause of obstruction, including congenital absence of the vas (CAV) or damage related to hernia repair: the length of residual epididymis in CAV determines the frequency of SpAbs; thus, when only a small residual head portion is present, SpAbs do not occur, indicating the important role of the epididymis in the generation of SpAbs in obstructive disorders;

(2) Blunt testicular trauma: when severe, this process is readily explainable on the basis of destruction of testicular architecture; however, the threshold for such trauma to permit SpAb production is unknown; it is possible that even minor and/or repetitive sporting trauma is sufficient;

(3) Testicular biopsy: evidence exists for a causal role for open biopsy, while needle-biopsy data are inconsistent, presumably because it is less traumatic;

(4) Orchitis or acute epididymitis;

(5) Genital tract infection appears to promote the generation of SpAbs: reports of an association between asymptomatic *Chlamydia* infection and SpAbs are available; the mechanism by which coexistent infections promote SpAb production is unclear; assessment for infection and appropriate antibiotic therapy is indicated if SpAbs (particularly IgA class) are detected.

Despite these known risks, many men presenting with SpAbs have no discernable risk factors, indicating that either they have gone unnoticed or other factors are operating. Interestingly, SpAbs are significantly associated with antithyroid microsomal antibodies, suggesting a genetic tendency to autoimmunity in some men. Reduced T lymphocyte-inhibitory activity in the seminal plasma of men with SpAbs has been suggested to contribute to their generation.

Functional consequences

It is clear that SpAbs may affect a wide range of sperm functions, but it is perplexing why these effects are not consistently seen in all men with similar levels of SpAbs. The variable expression of the following antifertility effects strongly suggests the presence of specific antigen–antibody interactions, leading to variable patterns of fertility impairment.

Sperm motility and cervical mucus interaction

SpAbs on the sperm surface can lead to agglutination in seminal plasma, which is apparent during routine semen analysis. Reduced motility featuring a 'shaking' and poorly progressive pattern can also be seen. However, an impairment of sperm penetration of cervical mucus correlates best with a reduction in fertility. The prevalence of motile sperm in cervical mucus following intercourse (the postcoital test) is significantly lower in SpAb-positive compared with SpAb-negative patients, as are the prospects of natural pregnancy. The localization of SpAbs to the sperm equatorial segment and the presence of the IgA class of SpAbs correlate with more marked fertility impairment. In practical terms, the likely impact of SpAbs on cervical mucus penetration is best evaluated in cross-over studies, where patient sperm are tested against healthy/fertile donor cervical mucus, while the female patient's cervical mucus is tested against healthy/fertile donor sperm.

Sperm vitality

Reduced sperm survival *in vitro* as a result of cytotoxic SpAbs has been reported. Complement is normally absent from the seminal plasma, although it might gain access to this compartment as a result of an injury. On the other hand, complement-dependent neutrophil-mediated sperm cytotoxicity has been reported in the female genital tract.

Sperm–oocyte interaction

Many aspects of this complex interaction can be impaired. SpAbs can impair sperm binding to the zona pellucida manifesting in a reduction in fertilization rates in conventional IVF. SpAbs can also inhibit sperm capacitation, as their addition to normal sperm impairs spontaneous and induced acrosome reactions. A reduction in zona pellucida penetration has been reported. Finally, an inhibition of sperm–oocyte fusion may be related to antibodies directed against antigens on the inner acrosomal membrane which become exposed after the acrosome reaction.

Post-sperm-binding events

It has been suggested that male-derived SpAbs might impair fertilization and embryonic development. However, recent data from ICSI treatments do not support this contention.

Diagnostic approaches

Many methods have been described for the detection of SpAbs; however, none has achieved universal acceptance as the gold standard. Ideally, a testing method would be well standardized and be both quantitative and specific in its detection of SpAbs directed to sperm antigens of established biological relevance. Unfortunately, in the absence of knowledge about the biologically significant sperm antigens, such a test does not exist. Rather, current methods detect immunoglobulin isotypes (IgG, A or rarely M) and, as such, are therefore limited.

SpAbs can be detected either attached to sperm (direct test) or in biological fluids (indirect test) such as serum, seminal or female genital tract fluids. The detection of SpAb binding directly to sperm is preferable, as the results of indirect tests are of less certain biological significance and subject to high assay variability. The two most popular commercial methods available are the immunobead test (IBT) and the mixed agglutination reaction (MAR).

In brief, the IBT utilizes polyacrylamide beads coated with murine IgG to human IgG, M and A, which are incubated with fresh motile sperm (direct test) or with normal donor sperm preincubated with patient fluids (serum or seminal plasma, indirect test). The strengths of the IBT are that the type of Ig, the percentage of sperm with beads attached and their location (head, midpiece, tail) can be quantified. Reagent costs, time and non-specific binding are difficulties.

The latter can arise as a result of the use of excessively high serum concentrations in the indirect test. Testing deportation is also impaired if the threshold for positivity is set too low (e.g. 20% labeling); most experienced authors set the threshold of likely biological significance at > 50% binding. Finally, it is believed that SpAbs directed only to the sperm tail tips are of dubious biological significance. Thus, it is incorrect to regard 80% tail-tip-only binding as biologically equivalent to 80% head and other sperm components; aggregating such subjects under one diagnostic umbrella will confound attempts to show relevance of the IBT test in populations.

The MAR test method uses latex beads or red blood cells labeled with human IgG, M or A, which are core-incubated with viable sperm following which anti-human Ig is added to cause agglutination with the sperm. Comparisons between IBT and MAR generally show a good correlation, although differences in sensitivities have been alleged. A raft of other tests (including enzyme-linked immunoassay or ELISA, flow cytometry, complement-mediated sperm immobilization) have not gained wide acceptance.

No diagnostic algorithm exists which relates the titer and location of SpAbs to known antigens that can be used, along with conventional semen and sperm mucus parameters, to provide the couple and the clinician with an evidence-based prediction of natural success. However, data showing that strongly positive SpAb results are associated with impaired fertility for both the MAR and IBT tests exist.

So what place does SpAb testing have in clinical practice? Given the lack of safe and effective treatment to reduce the impact of SpAbs on natural fertility, the primary purpose of testing is to provide advice to the couple about the likely cause of their disability and to facilitate timely referral to assisted reproductive technologies. However, owing to the imperfect nature of all current tests, abnormal results can only be considered advisory. Thus, while a poor mucus penetration test result is certainly an adverse finding for natural fertility, it does not exclude this possibility. When consulting with a couple in whom, for example, the IBT shows 90% of sperm with IgG and IgA on sperm head and tails, decisions about moving to assisted reproduction are also to be based on other biological (female partner's age and fertility) and subjective parameters (e.g. the desire for rapid outcome).

Management of male immunological infertility

There are three basic approaches to management: the removal of SpAbs to restore sperm function; reduction of SpAb production with immunosuppression; and assisted reproduction, specifically ICSI. Of these, safety and efficacy criteria strongly support the third approach.

Sperm antibody removal

Rapid washing of fresh sperm out of seminal plasma does not reduce SpAb load, i.e. they attach prior to ejaculation. Methods to reduce the prevalence of SpAb-positive sperm in the insemination sample (magnetic beads, washing, protease treatment) have been explored. Unfortunately, despite some success in reducing antibody load on sperm, data supporting improved fertility outcomes are lacking.

Immunosuppression

Immunosuppressive therapy with high doses of glucocorticoids, cyclically or continuously for 4–6 months, has been shown to improve pregnancy prospects in couples with severe sperm autoimmunity. Significant side-effects are frequent, and, although most are reversible, the rare septic necrosis of the hip is an irreversible and catastrophic outcome. Glucocorticoid treatment is not recommended as first-line treatment except under unusual circumstances, e.g. religious objection to IVF.

Assisted reproductive techniques

Intrauterine insemination

SpAbs are negatively correlated with success rates using intrauterine insemination (IUI). However, IUI has been advocated for mild to moderate sperm autoimmunity. However, few properly powered trials comparing IUI with natural well-timed intercourse have been conducted, and overall the data are not impressive. Thus, an early recourse to IVF/ICSI is warranted if IUI fails.

Assisted reproduction

Conventional IVF success rates are negatively impacted upon by SpAbs, presumably as a result of impairment of key sperm–egg interactions. The direct injection of isolated sperm into the oocyte cytoplasm circumvents all known adverse effects of SpAb on male fertility. Fertilization rates are no different from those seen using ejaculated sperm without SpAbs. Also, despite accessions to the contrary, SpAbs do not adversely affect post-fertilization and embryonic development nor increase pregnancy wastage. The excellent success rates with ICSI and its increasing availability have resulted in it becoming the first-line treatment for male immunological infertility.

A consequence of the success of ICSI has been a reduction in research efforts aimed at understanding the basis of SpAbs. Such a reduction of basic research is lamentable, as understanding the origin and relevance of specific antibody–antigen interactions provides two areas of benefit. First, it would supply better data on the natural history of male immunological infertility, which would assist in patient counseling. Second, such data may give key leads in the development of immunological methods for male contraception (see Chapter 3.4).

3.4 Immunocontraceptive vaccines

THE CASE FOR NOVEL AND MORE EFFECTIVE CONTRACEPTIVES

Despite the pill, male and female condoms, the Mirena® interauterine system (IUS) and other highly effective methods of contraception, the world's population continues to rise inexorably: in the 70 years between 1860 and 1930, the human population doubled to 2 billion, and in the next 70 it tripled, reaching the 6 billion mark on 12 October 1999. Even if fertility were to decline from its current rate of 3.3 to less than 2.5 children per woman, the global population would still increase to the anticipated 19 billion by the year 2100 and 28 billion by 2150. The human dimension of this predicament is made more acute by the fact that, at present, 95% of the population growth is in developing countries, and by that reckoning more than 80% of the world's population will be located in developing countries by the end of the century. There are also immediate arguments for more effective contraceptives: it is estimated that 210 million pregnancies occur worldwide each year, of which 38% are unplanned, and 22% (46 million) are terminated. Although the rates of pregnancy termination in the developed world remain high (23% of all US pregnancies are terminated, compared with the global figure of 22%), the impact of pregnancy termination differs depending on the economy. Thus, a woman having a pregnancy termination in Africa is 7000 times more likely to die from complications of the termination than her counterpart in, say, Canada (680 per 10 000 compared with 0.1 per 100 000).

There is, undoubtedly, an urgent need for more effective, more readily available and cheaper contraceptives than are currently available. The answer does not appear to lie in developing a yet more potent pill with fewer side-effects, nor a more effective intrauterine device (IUD) (the Mirena IUS is already as effective as sterilization) with cost implications, nor a cheaper condom, as both the male and the female condoms have not been universally acceptable where they are needed most. Perhaps the answer will ultimately lie with immunology. Just under 29 years ago (on 26 October 1977), WHO was able to announce eradication of the smallpox virus, thanks to effective global immunization programs. It is not totally unrealistic to draw analogies between immunization programs for infectious disease, and potential immunological interventions to control the world's population. Immunization is a modern miracle that saves more lives every day than any other medical intervention. The same principle could be applied to the development of effective contraception to control the world's population, to balance numbers against the available resources.

ATTRIBUTES OF A CONTRACEPTIVE VACCINE, AND POTENTIAL CHALLENGES OF DEVELOPING ONE

It is instructive and interesting to speculate on what the attributes of an ideal contraceptive vaccine might be. At the very least, the ideal contraceptive vaccine should possess the following:

(1) Safety, free from side-effects, and should therefore be directed against antigens unique to the reproductive system;

(2) Efficacy, ideally being at least as effective, if not better, than equivalent available methods – not difficult to achieve in principle especially in the Third World where women may have no access to contraceptives at all;

(3) Long-lasting, but reversible effects: the need for frequent boosters might compromise compliance, but the effects must either wear off within an acceptable time, or an 'antidote' must be available if they are to be used by women who might wish to have more children;

(4) Affordability, especially to the developing world where the need is greatest; for the developing-world setting, the delivery of vaccines should be facilitated by the fact that most developing countries possess a service infrastructure for the delivery of vaccines against disease into which a contraceptive vaccine could be incorporated.

The human being is a highly outbred species, characterized by considerable genetic diversity and extremely variable immunological responses to any given antigen. Since reliability is a major prerequisite for any contraceptive vaccine, such variability would be a major obstacle to the development of vaccines against pregnancy. Contraceptive vaccines should provide complete protection against pregnancy for a definable period of time. However, because of the inherent variability in responsiveness between individuals, it is likely that the administration of a contraceptive vaccine would have to be linked with an antibody-monitoring program to determine when booster injections might be necessary to maintain the contraceptive effect. Such monitoring programs would make the cost, convenience and feasibility of the approach difficult, if not unattainable, particularly in developing countries. Moreover, there is no compelling evidence that adequate antibody titers can be achieved in reproductive tract secretions to suppress such key biological events as sperm–egg recognition or blastocyst implantation. Additional difficulties, again especially relevant to the developing world include the likelihood that a significant proportion of the population may be immunologically compromised, rendering it difficult to predict the responsiveness of these individuals to any given vaccine.

The issue of reversibility is of paramount importance, since the basic premise on which most contraceptives are used is that when and if a couple should wish to embark on a pregnancy they should be able to do so. If reversibility cannot be guaranteed then a vaccine might not be acceptable to most couples, except those whose families are complete and who would then use the vaccine as a means of securing non-surgical sterilization.

The logistical problems are immense and the goal still elusive, but significant progress has been and continues to be made towards the development of effective contraceptive vaccines, although no such vaccine is as yet on the shelf, but still at the research and/or clinical trial stage. In the following section the current status of these research directions is discussed.

POTENTIAL ANTIGENIC TARGETS FOR CONTRACEPTIVE VACCINES

To date, the development of contraceptive vaccines has been targeted at three groups of potential antigens as follows:

(1) Sperm surface antigens;

(2) The zona pellucida;

(3) Implantation-associated antigens.

Sperm surface antigens

The idea of developing a contraceptive vaccine based on sperm surface antigens dates back to 1932, when Baskin showed that it was possible to induce sustained infertility in women by actively immunizing them with their husband's semen. Baskin was issued with a US patent for 'a non-specific spermatotoxic vaccine' in 1937, but ethical restrictions prevented further development of the approach. More recently, passive and active immunization trials have been conducted using more defined antigen preparations in animal models to determine the true potential of the spermatozoon as a target for immunocontraception. Since Baskin's time, considerable effort has been devoted to the identification of seminal antigens that might be used as the basis for a contraceptive vaccine. The concept of a fertility-regulating vaccine is also supported by a large volume of clinical data suggesting that occasional cases of human infertility are associated with the presence of antisperm antibodies (see Chapter 3.3). Since these patients appear to suffer no consequences of their immunity other than infertility, the development of a safe, effective vaccine targeting the spermatozoon should be feasible. Clearly, further development in this field will depend upon a detailed, molecular characterization of the sperm surface in order to identify antigens that are continuously expressed on the surface of the spermatozoon from the moment of ejaculation, and are antigenic, unique and capable of fixing complement, also important aspects of sperm function.

The development of the monoclonal antibody (MAb) has been a powerful tool, since it has allowed the identification of individual epitopes on the sperm surface or in semen. An example of such an epitope is PH-20, a sperm surface hyaluronidase for which homologs have been found in a wide variety of species, including the human. Contraceptive efficacy has been clearly demonstrated in both male and female guinea pigs. Male guinea pigs are particularly sensitive to PH-20, since only 5 mg of this protein can induce infertility in these animals. In human spermatozoa this antigen is localized on the outer surface of the plasma membrane overlying the acrosome, where it expresses the hyaluronidase activity necessary to facilitate sperm passage through the cumulus mass to the surface of the zona pellucida. Unfortunately, the infertility observed in male guinea pigs following the induction of immunity against PH-20 was associated with the induction of experimental autoimmune orchitis. Whether this orchitis is peculiar to guinea pigs or would be obtained in other species upon injection with purified or recombinant PH-20 remains to be ascertained, but is obviously a major concern with potential use in humans. Another guinea pig sperm antigen, fertilin (previously known as PH-30), resulted in complete fertility block after active immunization, although the incidence of orchitis was not assessed. However, no functional homolog of PH-30 appears to exist in humans, and therefore this particular molecule may not be a candidate for contraceptive vaccine development in humans.

Clearly, the process of sperm—oocyte fusion is central to fertility, and therefore a logical target for fertility regulation. Resolving the molecular mechanisms that drive this process is critical if it is to be a target for vaccine development. In this context, recent data indicating that nitric oxide is in some way involved in programming the sperm surface for fusion with the oocyte, and has a possible role in mediating the adhesion process, provide direction for future studies. Similarly, analysis of the molecular mechanisms responsible for controlling the sperm—zona interaction should produce potential candidates for contraceptive vaccine development. Characterization of human sperm surface antigens is still in its infancy, although several candidate molecules have already shown promise *in vivo*.

Sperm surface antigens could be developed as contraceptive vaccines in the male as well as the female. Clearly, clinical data support the general concept that anti-sperm antibodies could have a contraceptive effect in the male. The challenge will be to develop immunization protocols capable of generating local immune responses in the epididymis or, possibly, the secondary sexual glands, of sufficient intensity to compromise the function of millions of spermatozoa. Suppressing the function of the small population of spermatozoa that reach the site of fertilization in the female will always be a more straightforward proposition than targeting the large number of spermatozoa being continuously generated in the male reproductive tract. For this reason, antisperm vaccines are more likely to be developed for the control of fertility in the female rather than in the male.

The zona pellucida

The zona pellucida plays a key role in the initial stages of fertilization, in particular sperm—egg recognition, when the spermatozoa are induced to undergo the acrosome reaction. Given the uniqueness of the zona pellucida (in particular the ZP3 gene) and its central role during the early stages of fertilization, this molecule has been a clear target for the immunological control of fertility. It has been shown that transgenic mice that do not possess a zona pellucida because the ZP3 gene has been deleted are infertile. Studies conducted largely in the mouse have established that ZP3 is the zona glycoprotein responsible for both sperm—egg recognition and induction of the acrosome reaction.

It has been conclusively demonstrated that antibodies raised against ZP3, or recombinant peptides based upon this molecule, are capable of blocking fertilization *in vitro* in primates, including the human. It has also been widely documented that

109

the induction of active immunity against ZP3 will produce long-term infertility *in vivo* in a variety of species, including primates.

A major drawback of an anti-ZP3 vaccine has been the clear observation in marmoset monkeys that, although long-lasting infertility has been induced by actively immunizing with porcine ZP3, the infertility is invariably associated with a loss of ovarian function, characterized by a loss of primordial follicles from the ovary. Significantly, it often took more than a year for the ovarian pathology to appear in these marmoset studies. Thus, it is possible that in other primate trials where these side-effects have not been reported, the follow-up period may not have been extended for a sufficiently long period of time. It has been shown that the side-effects cannot be due to impurities in the antigen preparation, because they were also seen when recombinant proteins were used as the immunogen. Hence, reports indicating that recombinant zona vaccines can be used to reduce fertility in primates without eliciting ovarian dysfunction should be treated with caution until long durations of exposure have been assessed. Further progress in the development of zona pellucida vaccines can only be made when the ovarian pathology observed following the induction of immunity can be overcome. The challenge remains very much within the domain of the immunologist, since most evidence points to the possibility that a cytotoxic T cell response mediates the loss of the primordial follicles. However, the exact pathological mechanisms have yet to be elucidated. There are indications that the epitopes recognized in the unwanted effects are different from those recognized in the contraceptive effects, so that eradication of these epitopes from the vaccine may provide a solution. However, an alternative explanation for the ovarian pathology is that the loss of primordial follicles reflects the accelerated, futile recruitment of these cells into the growing follicle population, as the latter are eliminated due to the action of anti-ZP antibodies. This would explain the lag period between the induction of immunity and collapse of ovarian function. Yet another possibility is that a significant proportion of primordial follicles express low levels of ZP3, and that bound antizona antibodies might destroy the ovarian follicles by complement fixation. If either of the two latter explanations is correct, it would be difficult to imagine how an antizona vaccine could be developed that was not associated with severe side-effects of the type described.

Implantation-associated antigens

Human chorionic gonadotropin (hCG) is the hormone that signals the presence of the embryo to the maternal endocrine system, and has been an obvious potential target for contraceptive vaccine development. Indeed developments in this area have been most promising. hCG is secreted by the trophoblast of the implanting human blastocyst and passes in the maternal circulation to the ovary, where it serves to stimulate the continued production of progesterone by the corpus luteum. Thus, the embryo prevents the cyclical demise of the corpus luteum that precipitates menstruation. In principle, the induction of immunity against hCG should lead to a sequence of normal, or slightly extended, menstrual cycles during which any pregnancies would be terminated at around the blastocyst stage of development. The elegance of this approach is emphasized by its potential reversibility. The administration of a long-acting progestin over that critical period of time when the conceptus is dependent on the corpus luteum as a source of progesterone should prevent the contraceptive effect. However, the fact that such a vaccine would effectively function as an early abortifacient would be likely to render it unacceptable to some, such as the Roman Catholic Church, which opposes the intrauterine contraceptive device for the same reasons.

hCG is very similar in structure to the pituitary gonadotropin LH. These hormones consist of two subunits: the α subunit is identical in the two molecules, but the β subunit is identical for a short sequence of 37 amino acids at the carboxy-terminal of hCG. The development of immunogens to generate antibodies against hCG has therefore had to take account of this similarity. In order to minimize the immunological cross-reactivity with LH, candidate vaccines have been developed which are based on synthetic peptides representing the hCG-specific sequence, conjugated to immunogenic carriers such as diphtheria or tetanus toxoid. Vaccines incorporating the carboxy-terminal peptide (CTP) coupled to diphtheria toxoid have been used in phase I clinical trials and have been shown to produce significant antibody titers in the absence of any detectable side-effects. The antibody titers were thought to be adequate to neutralize the biological activity of hCG, although definitive proof that vaccination against this peptide will result in a contraceptive effect has not yet been achieved.

One of the major problems with CTP is its poor immunogenicity. Even when the antibody responses to this peptide reached an adequate titer, they were found to be too short-lived to be clinically useful. An alternative approach to developing powerful immunological responses to hCG has been to use the entire β subunit as the immunogen, rather than the C-terminal peptide. Initial studies were based on conjugation of the β subunit to tetanus toxoid. Clinical trials with these reagents demonstrated that it was feasible to raise antibodies against hCG and that the response was reversible and free from any harmful side-effects. The most significant shortcoming of this approach was that the antibody responses were variable from recipient to recipient, with the result that the poorest responders would not have experienced a contraceptive effect, given the low titers of anti-hCG antibodies obtained. The immunogenicity of the β subunit has been enhanced by the generation of hybrid hCG molecules, in which the β subunit of hCG is linked to the α subunit of ovine LH. Such hybrids have been found to induce the formation of conformational antibodies with greater biological activity than that of the isolated β subunit. Phase I clinical trials resulted in the generation of high anti-hCG antibody titers, with high avidity and enhanced bioactivity. Recently, a phase II efficacy trial has been completed with a heterospecific antigen in sexually active women of proven fertility. Immunization with the vaccine prevented pregnancy providing that antibody titers were above a certain critical threshold.

At present, the hCG vaccines appear to be free of adverse side-effects, even in the case of vaccines incorporating the entire β subunit of hCG, which clearly generates antibodies against LH. There has been no evidence of autoimmune reactions at the level of the pituitary gland and, somewhat surprisingly, no evidence of interference with normal menstrual cycle regularity. However, unexpected cross-reactivity has been observed against pancreatic islet cells with antibodies raised against the carboxy-terminal of the β subunit. Long-term *in vivo* studies will be needed to determine whether such cross-reactivity is significant. Where such studies have been conducted in non-human primates, the results have been very encouraging, even when the immunization protocols have involved the long-term induction of hyperimmunity against the β subunit of LH.

SUMMARY

The search for safe, effective, reversible and cheap contraceptives must continue unabated, and immunological approaches in the form of vaccines offer exciting possibilities. The most promising candidate antigens appear to be those that have the potential to interfere with two biological processes that are fundamental to the reproductive process, fertilization and maternal recognition of pregnancy. Our rudimentary understanding of the molecular mechanisms that control fertilization has hampered progress, but the zona pellucida glycoproteins may prove to be useful targets. Candidate sperm antigens will no doubt emerge as our understanding of sperm cell biology improves. Anti-hCG vaccines are already well advanced and certain formulations have entered phase III clinical trials. The technology underpinning vaccine development is constantly being developed, and innovations such as the use of cytokines or novel adjuvants to drive selective induction of specific classes of the immune response and the introduction of DNA vaccines are certain to impact upon the immunocontraception field. Safety and efficacy are key concerns that must be addressed during the vaccine engineering process. For example, the clinical consequences of immune responses below the threshold efficacy level will have to be investigated. For vaccines targeting the maternal recognition of pregnancy, the long term impact of 'failed' contraception on the fetus and child will also need to be taken into account. A major problem and challenge in the development of immuno-contraceptive vaccines is posed by the inherent interindividual variability in immune responsiveness. Such variability is bound to have a major impact on the predict-ability and the reliability of the vaccine regardless of the antigen being targeted.

4

The immune system and cancer

INTRODUCTION

Human papilloma viruses (HPV) are familiar to all gynecologists, as some types (6, 11 and their relatives) are predominantly associated with benign anogenital warts or condylomata, while other types (the high-risk types – 16, 18, 31, 33, 35, 45) are associated with anogenital cancers and intraepithelial lesions, particularly of the cervix. HPV are ubiquitous, and population-based serological studies show that most people who have been sexually active have antibodies to HPV, indicating that their immune system has encountered HPV at some point. Yet cervical cancer is relatively uncommon – there are only approximately 4000 new cases of invasive disease in the UK annually. It has tempted some to suppose that those women who develop precancer or cancer of the cervix are the ones who have encountered the high-risk types, while the rest have come across only low-risk HPV. This is, however, unlikely to explain the full picture. The general assumption is that there is some ill-defined immunological defect (perhaps at the local level, rather than a generalized defect) in those women who develop cancer, but the defect has yet to be defined. The notion of an 'immunosurveillance system' against cancer is widely believed, but whether it exists, and its nature, are subjects of debate and speculation. The link with the concepts regarding survival of the fetal allograft are clear enough: a cancer cell has undergone a transformation such that it should no longer be regarded as 'self', and presumably this is why cancer does not occur more frequently; the immunosurveillance system detects the 'non-self' cancer cells and destroys them, but as with any system, either the cancer cells develop ways of circumventing the 'immunological guards', or the latter become less efficient, or less energetic, allowing cancers to develop – which might explain why cancers are more common with increasing age! Many will have heard of cancer-related genes, and the gene p53 is known by many without an appreciation of what it is and its role in cancer. This chapter explores cancer and the immune system, with particular emphasis on gynecological malignancy.

WHY CELLS BECOME CANCEROUS: THE GENETIC BASIS OF ONCOGENESIS

It is highly plausible, and there is ample evidence to back this notion, that cancer arises when mutations occur in the genes of a normal cell. Within a cell, there are a group of genes called *proto-oncogenes* which serve an important function of growth and proliferation. However, if such genes undergo a mutation, or are switched on at an inappropriate time or at too high a level, cells that should not proliferate may be induced to do so, giving rise to a potential cancer cell. Mutations are of course very frequent and common events within cells, and as with most biological systems, there are built-in protective genes, the *anti-oncogenes*, whose products detect mutations in the proto-oncogenes, and trigger programmed cell death (apoptosis) in such cells before they become overtly cancerous. A well-know example of an anti-oncogene is p53, already mentioned in the 'Introduction'. Its crucial role in preventing cancer is such that it has been referred to as the 'guardian of the genome': when mutations have occurred, p53 will sense this and stop the cells proliferating until repair occurs if the mutations are limited, or trigger apoptosis if the mutations are extensive. But if proto-oncogenes mutate and the cell acquires the potential for cancer, and by chance anti-oncogenes also mutate so that the cell cannot defend itself against the activated proto-oncogenes, then a cancer may arise. Indeed, in most human cancers, p53 can be shown to be inactivated due to mutations. In experimental settings, mice that have been genetically modified so that they possess a mutant p53 are significantly more likely to develop cancers compared with their non-mutant counterparts. Since it is likely that multiple mutations are required before cancer can develop, and since it is likely to take a long time before a cell can accumulate sufficient mutations to become cancerous, this might explain why cancers occur most frequently in the old.

THE TRANSITION FROM NORMALITY TO CANCER

Although cancer is such a dreadful disease, in reality most cancers are rare, and this testifies to the effectiveness of the defenses against cancer, as well as the obstacles that a potential cancer cell must overcome before it can become full-blown cancer. For example, a potential cancer cell needs to overcome or escape the growth control mechanisms that normally keep cell proliferation in check. If a cell acquires a number of mutations, p53 can usually be relied upon as described above, and this is probably the way in which the vast majority of cancers are prevented. In addition, any potential tumor needs to establish an adequate blood supply in order to support and sustain its proliferation beyond a size of some two millimeters, since no cell can thrive in the body if at a distance greater than two millimeters from a blood vessel. In order to establish a blood supply, the potential tumor mass must be able to secrete molecules (angiogenic factors) that recruit new blood vessels into the growing mass. Since most cancer cells cannot do this, most growths remain small. Occasionally, a potential cancer cell acquires additional mutations which confer the ability to secrete angiogenic factors and thus to recruit new blood vessels. In this way the tumor can become large, but such a tumor may grow slowly, and therefore remains largely benign. Full-blown malignant potential is acquired when the cells undergo further mutations, acquiring the ability to secrete enzymes which can break down the membranes and structures that separate the growth from the bloodstream, allowing the cancer cells to metastasize.

SPONTANEOUS VERSUS VIRUS-ASSOCIATED CANCERS

The example of a virus-associated cancer has already been given in the 'Introduction': cancer of the cervix and its association with HPV. But the vast majority of human tumors are spontaneous, because they arise when a single cell accumulates a collection of mutations that cause it to acquire the properties of a metastatic cancer cell. These mutations can result from errors that are made when cellular DNA is copied to be passed to daughter cells, or from the effect of carcinogens. Mutations can also be caused by radiation (including ultraviolet (UV) light) or by errors in recombination. While these mutations occur 'spontaneously', factors that can accelerate the rate of mutation include cigarette smoking, certain diets (e.g. fatty diets) and increased exposure to radiation. The virus-associated cancer could in fact be considered in part 'spontaneous' in that mutations caused by errors in DNA copying, carcinogens and radiation may also be involved; a viral infection acts as an additional accelerating factor, as appears to be the case with cervical cancer and HPV. Presumably, HPV viral proteins expressed in infected cervical epithelial cells can functionally inactivate anti-oncogenes such as p53. Following establishment of a chronic infection in liver cells, hepatitis B virus may eventually induce cancer if its viral proteins inactivate p53. The fact that only a small proportion of individuals who are virus-infected will develop cancer supports the notion that the virus does not itself cause cancer, but accelerates the process that leads to the development of cancer.

A ROLE FOR THE IMMUNE SYSTEM IN PREVENTING CANCER?

The section on the genetic basis of oncogenesis above makes clear that anti-oncogenes such as p53 play a critical role in dealing with potential cancer cells. But are conventional immune mechanisms involved too? There is direct and indirect evidence for involvement of the immune system. Immunosuppression seen in acquired immune deficiency syndrome (AIDS) victims or following chemotherapy is associated with an increased incidence of cancers such as lymphomas, leukemias and virus-associated cancers. Laboratory experiments have shown that natural killer (NK) cells from 'stressed' mice have a reduced *in vitro* capacity to kill tumor cells when compared with NK cells from non-stressed mice, while anecdotal evidence in humans links increased cancer risk to stress. But there are problems with these observations and assumptions. Why, for example, is there no increase in the incidence of the most common human cancers, the spontaneous tumors that are not of blood-cell origin? If stress can so profoundly affect the immune system to the extent of allowing cancers to 'break through', what is the nature of such stress, and why, for example, are cancers not more common during or after wars, when humans are subjected to extremes of both physical (e.g. food deprivation) and psychological (e.g. extreme fear for prolonged episodes) stresses? Returning to the laboratory, nude mice, which lack functional T cells, do indeed suffer more lymphomas and leukemias, but not more non-blood-cell cancers, than normal mice. There is of course a possibility that the immune system is involved in defense against some, but not all kinds of cancer, and the section below deals with speculation on how this might be accomplished.

NATURAL KILLER CELLS AND MACROPHAGES IN ANTICANCER SURVEILLANCE

In Chapter 1 it was explained that when macrophages are hyperactivated, they secrete tumor necrosis factor (TNF), and also express it on their surface. Many tumor cells express TNF receptors on their surface. When these receptors bind TNF, a signal is transmitted to the cancer cell to commit suicide (apoptosis). This can be demonstrated *in vitro* with some cancer cells, but not with others. It is now known that in situations were TNF can induce tumor cell death *in vivo* but not *in vitro*, in the former it does so by attacking the blood cells that feed the tumor, depriving the tumor of a blood supply and causing the tumor to undergo necrosis (hence the term 'tumor necrosis factor'). A practical example of therapeutic intervention where macrophages are likely to play a pivotal role in the elimination of cancer cells is the treatment of melanoma with bacillus Calmette–Guérin (BCG), an attenuated form of the bacterium that causes tuberculosis. BCG hyperactivates macrophages, so that a tumor injected with BCG becomes infiltrated with large numbers of macrophages which can destroy it. BCG is similarly used in the treatment of superficial bladder cancers, where success has been well documented. What remains an enigma is how the macrophages distinguish between a normal and a cancerous cell. However, parallels have been drawn with the macrophage's other role, namely the elimination (by phagocytosis) of aging or old red blood cells in the spleen. In this instance, macrophages distinguish old red cells because the latter express the fat molecule phosphatidyl serine, while young red cells do not. Some tumor cells also express phosphatidyl serine on their surfaces and may thus be recognized. The very fact that they are cancer cells may also mean that they express other molecules that are also recognized by macrophages, but which have yet to be identified.

NK cells are also thought to recognize tumor cells if the latter express unusual surface molecules, although the exact nature of these is ill-understood. The NK cells then employ two mechanisms to kill the cancer cell. First, they can poke a hole in the membranes of cancer cells using perforin. Second, they can secrete enzymes that induce apoptosis. NK cells can also express Fas ligand on their surfaces which, on binding the Fas protein on tumor cells, triggers apoptosis also. These mechanisms of cell killing are similar to those employed by cytotoxic T lymphocytes (CTLs) to kill virus-infected cells (see Chapter 1). *In vivo*, NK cells may kill cancer cells directly, or may co-operate with other cells by releasing enabling cytokines.

The combination of macrophages and NK cells in cancer surveillance would appear to have a number of advantages. NK cells on the one hand do not need to be 'activated' to kill, the recognition of the correct target structure on a cancer cell being sufficient. Moreover, NK cells can produce cytokines such as interferon-γ (IFN-γ) which can activate macrophages, which then produce cytokines such as TNF which in turn can hyperactivate NK cells! Both NK cells and macrophages are well placed in peripheral tissues where tumors are likely to arise – they are therefore local and on site, ready to attack any aberrant cell with cancer potential. Even more important, both cells recognize diverse targets, which means, unlike the T cell which will recognize only a highly specific major histocompatibility complex (MHC)–peptide combination (see Chapter 1) they are able to recognize the almost limitless range of products of the spontaneous mutations that lead to cancer. Finally, they work almost immediately, in contrast to cells of the acquired immune system that would require priming: they can attack mutated cells almost immediately.

SURVEILLANCE AGAINST VIRUS-ASSOCIATED TUMORS BY CYTOTOXIC T LYMPHOCYTES

The cellular and humoral interactions that occur in the acute phase of any virus infection have been described elsewhere (see Chapter 1). The end result of most of these interactions is complete eradication of virus and development of immunity to that particular virus based on the development of memory capacity. An infection with chicken-pox or rubella would be a good example of such a scenario. However, some viruses somehow manage to evade total eradication, and establish a latent infection. A good example of such a scenario for the gynecologist is infection with the HPV, which form a latent infection in some cells of the cervix. It is not known exactly how latent infections are maintained, but it is likely that the latently infected cells go on to become cancer cells, and it is certainly the case that all viruses that are cancer-associated are able to establish latent infections. Even more intriguing is the fact that the latently infected cells continue to shed viral proteins, and yet appear to be 'invisible' to the immune system. A possible mechanism is that the molecules that allow recognition by the immune system are down-regulated, and it has certainly been demonstrated in laboratory studies that expression of MHC class I molecules and the TAP transporter is down-regulated in cells infected with HPV. Whatever the mechanism, memory CTLs that recognize HPV antigens are unable to kill the latently infected cells. Presumably, the memory CTLs can still be reactivated if latently infected cells start to churn out large volumes of viral particles which begin to infect other cells. In this way, the latent infection is kept under control. This may be an explanation as to why humans who are immunosuppressed tend to have a high rate of virus-associated tumors – they lack the memory CTLs to keep latent infections at bay, and more cells acquire the latent infection and therefore raise the numbers of cells with the potential to become malignant. Thus, CTLs would appear to be ineffectual in surveillance against cancer from viruses that can establish latent infections.

SURVEILLANCE AGAINST SPONTANEOUS TUMORS BY CYTOTOXIC T LYMPHOCYTES

The concept of self-tolerance renders it difficult to conceive how naive T cells could be involved in immunosurveillance. Ordinarily, naive T cells circulate continuously through the blood, lymph and secondary lymphoid organs, but do not leave the circulation pattern to enter tissue where cancers may form. They would only do so after they had been activated. Thus, it is difficult to conceive how virgin T cells could ever 'see' tumor antigens expressed in tissues. There is, therefore, a serious conflict between the need to preserve tolerance of self (and avoid autoimmune disease) and the need to provide surveillance against tumors that arise, as most tumors do, in the tissues. In this instance, it would seem that tolerance wins.

Even if there was the possibility of a virgin T cell entering tissue by chance, for T cells to be activated, they must recognize their cognate antigen presented by MHC molecules, and they must also receive co-stimulatory signals. Since CTLs recognize antigens that are produced within a cell and presented by class I MHC, the tumor cell itself would have to present the tumor antigens. Even if this could happen, it seems unlikely that the tumor cell could also provide the co-stimulation required for activation, since it is not an antigen-presenting cell after all. Therefore, the more likely outcome of a virgin T cell entering tissue and recognizing tumor antigen is that the CTL itself will be anergized because the tumor cell cannot provide the co-stimulation that the CTL needs. This illustrates yet again the conflict between tolerance induction and tumour surveillance: T cells which recognize self-antigens in the tissues, but receive no co-stimulation, will be anergized or killed to prevent autoimmunity. But this renders CTLs unable to respond to tumor cells. Of course, the CTLs could be activated if a tumor cell metastasizes to a lymph node, but this would also suggest that the tumor is at an advanced stage, with individual cancer cells mutating rapidly and posing a major challenge for the CTLs, which may not be able to keep up with the mutations and fail to recognize the cancer cells, or deal with what must be a large tumor mass at this stage. In fact it is estimated that at least 15% of the tumors that have been examined have turned off expression of at least one of their MHC molecules. Further, in the tumor cell, genes that encode the LMP proteins or the TAP transporters can mutate, so that tumor antigens will not be efficiently processed or transported for loading on to class I MHC molecules. This high mutation rate is the tumor's greatest advantage over the immune system, and it can usually keep tumor cells one step ahead of surveillance by CTLs. Hence, when it occurs, CTL surveillance is probably a case of 'too little, too late'. Hence, CTLs are unlikely to provide serious surveillance against non-blood-cell, spontaneous tumors. It is possible that CTLs are useful against bloodcell cancers such as leukemia and lymphoma. After all, immunosuppressed humans and mice have higher frequencies of leukemia and lymphoma than do normal humans and mice. This suggests that there might be something fundamentally different about the way the immune system views tumors in tissues and organs versus the way it views blood cells that have become cancer cells. In contrast to cancer occurring in tissues, most blood-cell cancers are found in the blood, lymph and secondary lymphoid organs, where they come into contact with CTLs, which are passing through these areas all the time, i.e. the traffic patterns of cancer cells and virgin T cells actually intersect. Moreover, some cancerous blood cells actually express high levels of B7 (a co-stimulatory molecule) and, therefore, can provide the necessary co-stimulation. These properties of blood-cell cancers suggest that CTLs might provide surveillance against some of them. Unfortunately, this surveillance must be incomplete, because people still get leukemias and lymphomas.

SOME PRACTICAL CONSIDERATIONS

It is very attractive, and certainly plausible, to suppose that the immune system mounts some kind of surveillance against cancer. The potential role of NK cells and macrophages is described above, and is probably the important mechanism. CTLs do not seem to play a major role in immunosurveillance, especially for cancers in tissue. However, researchers have shown that CTLs from some cancer patients can kill tumor cells *in vitro*. There is therefore a potential for manipulating CTLs so that they can destroy cancer cells in patients. Early data using this approach are certainly promising. Immunological concepts in cancer are particularly important and applied in immunodiagnostics. For example, the oncogene HER-2/neu is an epidermal growth factor (EGF) receptor, characterized by an extracellular domain which protrudes beyond the cell membrane. In breast cancer, and also in some other cancers, up to 40% of tumors can be shown to overexpress HER-2/neu. The prognosis for patients whose tumors are HER-2/neu-positive is poor unless they are treated with a humanized monoclonal antibody (trastuzumab) raised against HER-2/neu which binds to the extracellular domain, blocking the ability of EGF to bind to it. Unlike other cancer therapies, trastuzumab is targeted specifically towards cells which overexpress HER-2/neu, resulting in a very low side-effects profile. This is presented as an example of the potential for immunology, in both diagnosis and treatment. The ultimate dream is the development of a tumor-specific antibody to which a drug or anticancer molecule can be attached, which can be given to patients whereupon it circulates in blood and tissues, targets tumors and eliminates them. This is not a pipe-dream!

THE IMMUNOBIOLOGY OF HUMAN PAPILLOMA VIRUS

For the gynecologist, HPV is an important virus, and its immunobiology warrants a more detailed discussion before this chapter ends. A number of key observations are central to an understanding of the potential role of the immune system in HPV infections:

(1) HPV infections are ubiquitous – most people who have engaged in sexual activity possess antibodies to HPV. But these antibodies appear to play no significant role in the maintenance of infection since disorders of humoral immunity do not result in increased susceptibility to HPV infections, although they may protect against reinfection.

(2) On the other hand, immunocompromised individuals (human immunodeficiency virus (HIV) or transplant patients on immunosuppressive drugs) show an increased incidence and progression of HPV infections. This illustrates a critical role for cell-mediated immune responses in the resolution and control of HPV infections.

(3) The vast majority of individuals who become infected with HPV clear the infection without overt clinical disease, while those who develop lesions, in most cases, mount an effective cell-mediated immune response which causes the lesions to regress.

A basic understanding of the natural history of HPV infection, the genomic structure of HPV and the infectious cycle is the key to understanding the pathogenesis and immunobiology of HPV infection.

The natural history of human papilloma virus infection

This is simple enough: transient infections are common and sexually transmitted; most are subclinical and resolve, and where lesions develop they are also self-limiting and regress; a very tiny minority of women develop persistent infections with focal high levels of DNA, and where the infection is with a high-risk HPV type, the infection may progress to cervical intraepithelial neoplasia, which in turn may progress to invasive carcinoma.

The genomic structure of human papilloma virus

There are in excess of 130 HPV genotypes. The DNA of more than 80 genotypes has now been sequenced, and there is an overall high degree of conservation of genomic organization. Figure 4.1 showing HPV 16 is illustrative of the genomic architecture. The HPV genome can be divided into three domains: a non-coding upstream regulatory region (URR) of approximately 1 kb, an early region with open reading frames (ORFs) E6, E7, E1, E2, E4 and E5 and a late region encoding two genes L1 (the major capsid protein) and L2 (the minor capsid protein). Table 4.1 describes the functions of the ORFs.

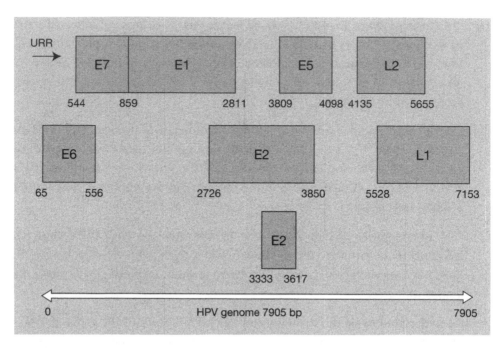

Figure 4.1 Genomic architecture of human papilloma virus (HPV) 16. Open reading frames (ORFs) are denoted as boxed areas shaded in color. Overlapping co-ordinates of the eight ORFs are indicated. URR, upstream regulatory region

Table 4.1 Functions of human papilloma virus (HPV) 16 open reading frames

L1	major capsid protein
L2	minor capsid protein
E1	helicase essential for viral DNA replication
E2	viral transcription factor binds E1 to facilitate initiation of viral DNA replication important in genome encapsidation
E4	interacts with cytoskeletal proteins, allows viral assembly
E5	weak transforming activity up-regulates growth factor receptor numbers
E6	immortalizes primary human keratinocytes in co-operation with E7 binds p53 and directs p53 degradation by ubiquitin-targeted proteolysis
E7	immortalizes primary human keratinocytes in co-operation with E6, transcriptase transactivator binds pRb with deregulation G1/S checkpoint in the cell cycle

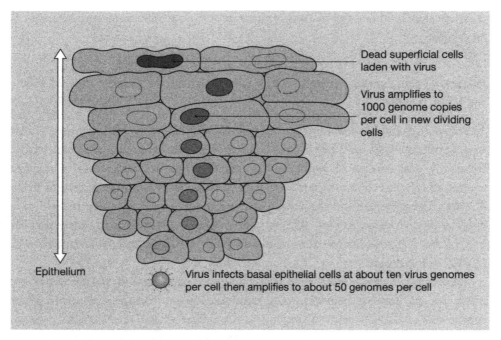

Figure 4.2 Replication cycle of human papilloma virus

Infectious cycle of human papilloma virus

Knowledge of the HPV infectious cycle has been limited by failure to develop an *in vitro* model, and the fact that papilloma viruses are highly species-specific. Although the sequence of events illustrated in Figure 4.2 is widely accepted as representing events in the infectious cycle, it has been deduced from animal studies and may not be entirely accurate.

Although the virus infects primitive basal keratinocytes, high-level viral expression of viral proteins and viral assembly occur only in the upper layers of squamous epithelia. Thus, infection and vegetative viral growth are absolutely dependent upon a complete program of keratinocyte differentiation. Since the time taken for the keratinocytes to undergo complete differentiation and desquamation is approximately 3 weeks, the replication cycle for HPV is at least 3 weeks, and in reality the period between infection and the appearance of lesions varies from weeks to months. This indicates that HPV can effectively evade the immune system. Since viral replication and assembly take place in the differentiating keratinocyte, a cell destined for death and desquamation far from the sites of immune activity, there is no cytolysis or cytopathic death. Thus, HPV infection does not elicit an inflammatory reaction, the immune system is not alerted and a potential for a chronic persistent infection is established.

Nature of the immune response to human papilloma virus: a critical role for CD4 T cells

The increased incidence and progression of HPV infection in HIV patients points to a significant role for CD4 T cells. This has been confirmed via several routes. Immunological studies of spontaneously regressing genital warts show a massive mononuclear cell infiltration into both stroma and epithelium, dominated by CD4 T cells. The cytokine profile within the regressing lesions is characteristic of a delayed-type hypersensitivity (DTH) Th1-biased response, with expression of mRNA for the pro-inflammatory cytokines IFN-γ, TNFα and the interleukin-12 (IL-12) p40 subunit.

Studies in animal models, especially canine oral papilloma virus infection, have confirmed the findings from the cross-sectional studies in humans with regard to the central role of CD4 T cells. However, it is not known which viral antigens provoke the response, although HPV E6 and E7 are likely to be strong candidates. The limited data available seem to suggest that there may be species differences in the viral antigens eliciting the immune responses.

With regard to cytotoxic T cell responses, again data are scanty. However, all evidence points to an important role for CTLs in the clearance of HPV infection. Both CD4 and CD8 cytotoxic effector cells are thought to be implicated. High-affinity HPV E7-specific CTLs have been shown to be rare in patients with carcinoma or high-grade cervical intraepithelial neoplasia (CIN), although they can be detected.

The humoral response to HPV does not appear to be important in clearing lesions, although it may play a role in preventing reinfection (at least in animals). Because of a lack of suitable antigenic targets for serological assays, studies of humoral immunity to HPV have had to rely on the use of virus-like particles (VLPs), and these have demonstrated humoral responses to the L1 capsid protein in both high- and low-risk virus infections. However, the assays are of low sensitivity, and the variable time interval between infection and seroconversion renders serum antibody responses rather useless for diagnostic purposes.

The future of human papilloma virus infection: vaccines

The limited knowledge of the nature of the immune response has not deterred attempts to develop vaccines against HPV. VLPs have been utilized as immunogens for prophylactic vaccinations, and clinical trials have already been conducted. Phase II clinical trials have shown that a vaccine against four common HPV types (16 and 18, which cause 70% of cervical cancer and high-grade cervical intraepithelial neoplasia; and 6 and 11, which cause 90% of anogenital warts) prevents the development of the related clinical disease. The incidence of persistent infection or disease 36 months following vaccination with an HPV L1 virus-like particle vaccine was 90% lower in the vaccinated women compared with those given placebo. Also very impressive was the finding that no cases of pre-cancerous cervical lesions or genital warts associated with the four HPV types developed in the vaccine group. Thus, HPV vaccination could substantially reduce the occurrence of disease in developing countries, while also cutting the costs linked to the management of abnormalities detected by screening in the developed world.

Overall, virtually all results of clinical trials of HPV vaccines are yielding highly promising results, and at least one vaccine is expected to be licensed for use in 2006. It has been suggested that a vaccine containing the seven most common HPV types could prevent about 87% of cervical cancers world-wide, with little regional variation.

All this good news notwithstanding, some epidemiologists have suggested that there are clinical, epidemiological and ethical questions that need to be addressed before the introduction of widespread vaccination programs. Some of their questions/concerns include the following:

- What benefits might vaccination confer on adults who are already infected with HPV?

- What proportions of cervical cancer and other HPV-related disease in a region or country are attributable to the HPV types targeted by the available vaccines?

- Will a vaccination program against a sexually transmitted infection prove acceptable to adolescents who are not yet sexually active, and to their parents?

- Should teenage boys be vaccinated, as well as teenage girls?

- How will a vaccination program affect current programs for cervical cancer screening, and how and when should screening change in response?

These and other issues are of vital importance, but given the scale of the problem, especially in the developing world, it is to be hoped that there will now not be any significant delay in licensing these critically important vaccines. The new International Finance Facility for Immunization should be used to speed the delivery of the vaccines to the developing world, where the need and benefits will be greatest.

5

Immunopathology in obstetric and gynecological practice

So far the immune system has been portrayed as 'the good guy', the great defender against intrinsic disease including malignancy, and extrinsic invaders such as infectious organisms. However, as with all biological systems, things can and do go wrong: diseases may arise because of genetic or acquired deficiencies in the immune system; the great defender may turn against self (autoimmune disease); the mechanisms that regulate the immune system may fail; or the immune system may work properly, but in the face of tricky or more aggressive customers the 'normal' response may in fact result in pathology. This chapter explores these issues.

IMMUNODEFICIENCY: GENETIC AND ACQUIRED

Genetic immunodeficiency

Perhaps the ultimate example of a genetic defect leading to profound immunological compromise is the severe combined immunodeficiency syndrome (SCIDS), but this is a rare condition. The patient lacks functional T and B cells, and is therefore unable to mount both humoral and cellular immune responses and cannot survive except in a germ-free environment. There are other examples of less extensive genetic defects, but in reality such defects are also very rare.

Acquired immunodeficiencies

Acquired immunodeficiencies are much more common. While they may be iatrogenic, such as immunosuppression induced during organ transplantation or as a result of chemotherapy, in the modern era the vast majority are a result of infection by the human immunodeficiency virus (HIV). This has turned out to be the scourge

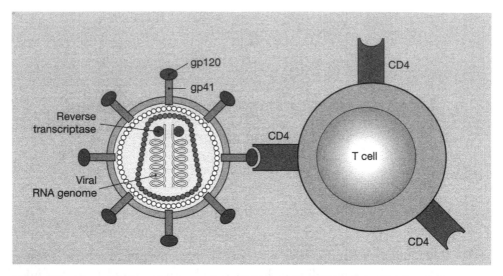

Figure 5.1 Human immunodeficiency virus (HIV) infectivity. HIV binds to CD4 T cells through its coat of glycoprotein gp120. Since CD4 is also expressed on the surface of cells of the macrophage lineage, they too can be directly infected by HIV. The viral protein gp41 then mediates fusion of the enveloped virus with the target cell, allowing the viral genome to enter the cell

of the 21st century, with more than 50 million people currently living with this infection, the vast majority in the developing world.

It is pertinent to explain briefly how HIV induces immunodeficiency. The HIV is an RNA virus which, after infecting a cell, is copied by an enzyme called reverse transcriptase to make a 'copy' DNA (cDNA). Next, the DNA of the cell is cut by an enzyme carried by the virus, and the viral cDNA is inserted into the gap in the cellular DNA, where it can remain in a latent state, unrecognizable by cytotoxic lymphocytes (CTLs). Later on the latent virus can reactivate and replicate, producing more virus particles which can then infect other cells. An important aspect in the virus' ability to evade the immune system is that the reverse transcriptase that copies the viral RNA shows a high degree of mutation – in other words, often the new viruses that are produced by an infected cell are different from the virus that originally infected the cell. This means that any previously initiated immune response may be useless against the new mutated virus, and thus the immune system may never keep pace with the rapidly mutating virus. Even worse is the fact that HIV specifically targets key cells of the immune system: when infecting a cell, HIV binds to the all important CD4 molecule, the co-receptor protein found on helper T cells, macrophages and dendritic cells. Thus, these cells either themselves become targets for destruction by CTLs (as they are now virus-infected), or are killed by the virus

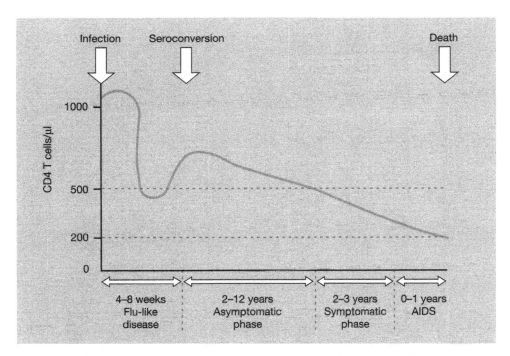

Figure 5.2 Typical course of infection with human immunodeficiency virus (HIV). Infection is followed by an acute flu-like febrile phase lasting some 4–8 weeks, with high viral titers in the blood, and development of anti-HIV antibodies (seroconversion). An adaptive immune response follows with restoration of CD4 T cell levels and control of the acute illness. But the virus is not eradicated and CD4 levels continue to fall. Opportunistic infections and other symptoms become most frequent as the CD4 T cell count falls, starting at around 500 cells per microliter. The symptomatic phase then ensues, culminating in death. AIDS, acquired immune deficiency syndrome

or have their function disrupted. Hence, the immunodeficiency seen in HIV-infected patients is a result of the destruction of helper T cells and antigen-presenting cells (Figure 5.1).

Thus, the key reasons that HIV is so successful and devastating (Figure 5.2) are as follows:

• Its ability to establish a latent infection that cannot be detected by CTLs

• Its high mutation rate meaning that it can effectively elude any CTLs and antibodies directed against it

• The fact that the virus specifically targets key cells of the immune system – helper T cells and antigen-presenting cells

The health, social and economic impact of HIV is clear for all to see. Despite billions of dollars being poured into research, in terms of understanding both the dis-

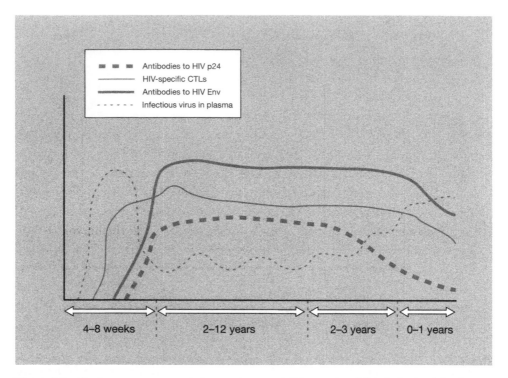

Figure 5.3 The immune response to human immunodeficiency virus (HIV). Following infection, an initial sharp rise in infectious virus provokes a cellular and humoral response, with a sharp fall in viral load, the maintenance of high levels of HIV-specific cytotoxic T lymphocytes (CTLs), and the production of antiviral antibodies. However, the virus is never completely eradicated, and despite high levels of CTLs and antibodies, CD4 T cell counts continue to fall. Eventually the levels of antibody and HIV-specific CTLs also fall, and viral load rises

ease process and the drugs and other therapeutic strategies, as yet there is no cure or vaccine of proven efficacy for this devastating virus. From the point of view of reproduction, a major tragedy is the vertical transmission of HIV. In the developed world, strategies including antiretroviral therapy during pregnancy, delivery by elective cesarean section, administration of antiretroviral medications to the neonate and avoidance of breast-feeding now mean that the rate of vertical transmission can be reduced to as low as 1–2%. In the developed world, the availability of a wide range of antiretroviral medications also means that the prognosis for HIV-infected individuals is rapidly changing for the better, and many people can now expect to survive in relatively good health for decades. Unfortunately this does not apply to the developing world, where the infection is now way beyond epidemic levels, and where scarce resources mean that those who most need treatment have no access to it (Figure 5.3).

AUTOIMMUNE DISEASE

Obstetricians will be familiar with systemic lupus erythematosus (SLE), rheumatoid arthritis and type I (insulin-dependent) diabetes (IDDM) as classic examples of autoimmune diseases that render pregnancies 'high risk'. SLE predisposes to major pregnancy wastage, with affected women experiencing recurrent miscarriages, intrauterine growth restriction and a high incidence of pre-eclampsia and intrauterine death. (Note that SLE should not be confused with the primary antiphospholipid syndrome, which is also associated with a major degree of pregnancy wastage, and which has some markers in common with SLE: see Chapter 3.1). Rheumatoid arthritis, on the other hand, offers a two-edged sword with regard to pregnancy. In the 1930s the surprising clinical observation that rheumatoid arthritis tended to undergo remission during pregnancy ultimately led to the discovery of cortisone, and the award of the Nobel Prize to Hench. It is now well known that a remarkable 75% of sufferers experience a remission during pregnancy, but a relapse within the first 3 months post-delivery is common. From a practical point of view, women with severe debility will encounter problems with child-rearing due to deformity of the upper limbs. Until the discovery of insulin, women with IDDM rarely achieved successful pregnancies. Now, in developed countries, the goal of obstetricians/diabetic physicians is to provide care to such women to a point where maternal and perinatal mortality and morbidity equates to that of women without IDDM. While this goal has been achieved in some European countries such as Germany and the Scandinavian countries, in the UK it has yet to be achieved.

An autoimmune disease implies that the extensive processes that normally preserve tolerance to 'self' (see Chapter 1) have somehow failed. But why does the immune system occasionally attack the very 'self' it is supposed to defend? Although we know a great deal about the pathophysiology of most of these diseases, such as identifying the autoantibodies that mediate the disease process, in fact at present no one really knows why an individual develops SLE or rheumatoid arthritis or type I diabetes: why antibodies to self-components should be formed. There are, however, clues in what we know about these diseases:

(1) First, there is often a strong familial predisposition, and this is true of all three examples of autoimmune diseases cited. In the case of type I diabetes, the inheritance of two particular types of class II major histocompatibility complex (MHC) genes increases the risk of developing diabetes 20-fold, and while SLE is in fact uncommon, it is not unusual for two sisters to develop the condition. Thus, genetic susceptibility is an essential requirement for the development of autoimmune disease.

(2) Second, it is well known that autoimmune diseases often follow microbial infections. The theory of 'molecular mimicry' has arisen from this observation whereby it is postulated that T or B cells which recognize certain microbial antigens are activated by the microbial invasion in the usual way, but that the receptors on these immune cells happen to cross-react with 'self' antigens. In Chapter 1, although the concept of one-antigen-one-receptor was widely espoused, a given T cell receptor (TcR) or B cell receptor (BcR) can usually recognize several antigens, but with varying affinities. Similarly, a given MHC molecule can present a large number of peptides that have the same general characteristics of binding motifs, hydrophobicity, length, etc. Thus, the potential for cross-reactivity exists: self-reactive lymphocytes are activated by a cross-reacting microbial antigen, and then cause damage to self even after the microbial invaders are eliminated.

Since BcRs and TcRs which recognize self-antigens have the potential to cross-react with multiple environmental antigens, it seems unlikely that a given autoimmune disease could be caused by a single environmental antigen. On this understanding, it is perhaps surprising that autoimmune diseases are not more common, or indeed more diverse. It is quite likely that activation of self-reactive lymphocytes is a common event, but that the vast majority are deleted by apoptosis or become anergic when they lack continuous restimulation. Thus, other factors must be operational for an autoimmune disease to progress. Current thinking is that inflammation plays an important role in the propagation of autoimmune disease, as local inflammatory cytokines produced in an area of inflammation will activate antigen-presenting cells (APCs) such as macrophages, which in turn will express the MHC and co-stimulatory molecules required to restimulate any self-reactive lymphocytes that might traffic into an area of inflammation where the self-antigen is expressed. But if there is no inflammation, or if the self-antigen is not expressed in the area of inflammation, the self-reactive lymphocyte will be deleted for lack of restimulation. This might explain why autoimmune diseases are in fact relatively rare.

To summarize, an autoimmune disease can only develop if the following three prerequisites are met:

(1) A genetic susceptibility: the possession of MHC molecules that can present self-antigens, and TcRs that recognize these self-antigens;

(2) An environmental trigger: a microbial invasion when TcRs that cross-react with self-antigens are activated (the concept of molecular mimicry);

(3) Reactivation of the self-reactive lymphocytes: a simultaneous inflammatory reaction in tissues where the self-antigen is expressed, so that APCs will be

activated and pick up the self-antigen to present to the self-reactive lymphocytes.

What is known of the immunopathology of the examples of autoimmune diseases cited above follows.

Systemic lupus erythematosus

This is a multisystem disorder which typically affects young women, commonly presenting with arthritis or arthralgia, although others may present with skin lesions (the classical red rash on the forehead and cheeks – giving the 'red wolf' appearance for which the disease is named), hair loss and pulmonary, renal, neurological (paralysis and convulsions) and hematological disease. A full description of the clinical presentation, laboratory findings and management is beyond the scope of this book (see 'Suggested reading' at the end of chapter 1). Owing to the high pregnancy wastage, women with SLE are best managed in tertiary centers with accumulated expertise and experience and the availability of multidisciplinary teams. Ideally, a woman should be assessed prior to pregnancy to optimize disease control, and pregnancy should be embarked upon during a quiescent phase. Any disease flares should be treated aggressively, and steroid therapy (prednisolone) with careful monitoring has been shown to be safe during pregnancy. The fetus is a patient too, who should be subjected to high surveillance with regular growth scans, Doppler blood flow studies and timely delivery when there is evidence of compromise (intrauterine growth restriction due to placental insufficiency is a common feature of SLE). Some newborns show transient features of SLE, and congenital heart block is a rare but well-recognized complication. With care in specialized centers, the prognosis for pregnancy outcome in women with SLE has shown dramatic improvement. Flares in the puerperium are not uncommon, and continued surveillance is therefore crucial.

From an immunological point of view, there appears to be a breakdown in both B and T cell tolerance that results in the production of IgG antibodies which recognize a wide range of self-antigens including DNA, DNA–protein complexes and RNA–protein complexes. Given the diversity of the autoreactive antibodies, it is hardly surprising that SLE should be a multisystem disorder.

The fact that the probability of identical twins both having SLE increases tenfold over the 2% probability seen in non-identical twins indicates a strong genetic component to the disease. Multiple MHC and non-MHC genes have been identified, each of which seems to increase slightly the probability that a person will contract SLE.

Two drugs that obstetricians and gynecologists will be very familiar with have been implicated in the initiation of SLE: hydralazine used in the treatment of hypertension in pregnancy, and minocycline, an antibiotic used as long-term treatment for acne. However, other drugs too have been implicated, including procainamide and D-penicillamine. No specific microbial infection has been associated with the initiation of SLE. Two animal models of SLE have suggested that defective apoptosis may play a role: mice that lack functional genes for Fas or Fas ligand exhibit SLE-like symptoms. Apoptosis triggered through Fas appears to have an important role in deleting autoreactive lymphocytes, which are then thought to cause disease when they are not deleted. It should be emphasized that human SLE is not associated with Fas deficiency, and other mechanisms are likely to be responsible.

Rheumatoid arthritis

This disease does not cause infertility or increased pregnancy wastage, and indeed the remarkable point has already been made above that there is a 75% remission rate in association with pregnancy. The significance of rheumatoid arthritis to reproductive immunobiology therefore lies in the high relapse rates in the puerperium, and in severely affected mothers with significant limb deformity, the difficulties they may encounter with independent child-rearing.

Rheumatoid arthritis is characterized by chronic inflammation of the joints. The exact mechanisms involved remain obscure, but there has been extensive research over the years, and the accumulated data have not only provided fascinating clues on causation, but also indicated directions in effective therapeutic interventions. A genetic predisposition exists, but the genes involved have yet to be identified. It is suspected that the bacterium that causes tuberculosis may be the environmental trigger in at least some cases of rheumatoid arthritis: mice injected with *Mycobacterium tuberculosis* suffer from inflammation of the joints and exhibit lesions not dissimilar to those seen in humans. One of the presumed targets of the autoimmune reaction in rheumatoid arthritis is a cartilage protein, and the quantum leap in understanding disease processes has been the finding that autoreactive T cells from rheumatoid arthritis patients recognize both the cartilage protein and a protein encoded by *M. tuberculosis*. Additional evidence suggests that under the direction of autoreactive helper T_h cells, macrophages infiltrate joints where they produce large amounts of tumor necrosis factor (TNF), which appears to mediate the inflammatory process that causes damage to the joints. IgM antibodies that recognize and bind to the crystallizable fragment (Fc) region of IgG antibodies are also present in the joints of individuals with rheumatoid arthritis, and these IgM–IgG antibody complexes additionally activate the macrophages that have entered the joints, further increasing the inflammatory reaction. The quantum leap that has been made with regard to treatment has been the demonstration that treatment of patients with anti-TNF antibodies results in considerable improvement: infliximab (anti-TNF antibody-based drug) is now a major component of the armamentarium in the treatment of rheumatoid arthritis.

Type I diabetes

This is an example of an organ-specific autoimmune disease. It is important in reproduction because poorly managed disease compromises pregnancy, and pregnancy itself affects disease management. Poorly controlled IDDM is associated with increased risk of congenital malformation, miscarriage, preterm birth, hypertension and birth trauma, as well as neonatal hypoglycemia. Insulin requirements fluctuate and tend to increase during pregnancy, and some diabetic lesions may progress more rapidly during pregnancy. However, optimal control during pregnancy, achieved by management by multidisciplinary teams comprising diabetologists, obstetricians, diabetic nurse specialists and midwives, as well as other specialists when required including renal physicians and ophthalmologists, reduces the risk of most if not all of these potential complications.

With regard to immunopathology, it is believed that in the initial phase, the insulin-producing β cells of the pancreas are attacked by autoreactive CTLs. Autoreactive B cells then produce antibodies targeted against the same cells which then mediate the chronic inflammation that contributes to the pathology of the disease.

The probability that both identical twins will have IDDM is estimated at 50%, suggesting a strong genetic susceptibility, but no environmental triggers have yet been identified. Since the antibodies to the β-cells are produced long before symptoms of the disease appear, surveillance of potential sufferers can be conducted by screening for antibodies in close relatives of patients with active disease.

Other autoimmune diseases

There are of course other diseases such as multiple sclerosis, myasthenia gravis, pemphigus vulgaris and Graves' disease, to name but a few. In some, such as Graves' disease, the autoreactive antibodies have been clearly described, while in others there are features of autoimmunity, but the pathophysiology remains largely obscure. Most of these other diseases have little, if any, impact on reproduction, and therefore are not explored in any detail here.

HYPERSENSITIVITY

Diseases may arise because of defects in regulation of the immune system, or when a normal immune response, in addition to the intended destruction of an antigen, results in tissue damage. Such immune reactions are grouped together under 'Hyper-sensitivity', and four main types of hypersensitivity reactions are recognized, described below with examples. A type V reaction has been proposed for the immunostimulation responses caused by some non-complement-fixing antibodies (e.g. thyroid stimulating immunoglobulins), but this category is not associated with immunological damage. It should be recognized that the four main types of reaction are not mutually exclusive and often coexist, involving a mixture of mechanisms.

Type I hypersensitivity reactions

Hay fever is the quintessential example of the 'allergies' that afflict up to 20% of the population. Other common allergic reactions include asthma, rhinitis and conjunc-tivitis. Even non-immunologists will be familiar with the basic concept of the aller-gic reaction – the release of histamine by mast cells upon stimulation by an appro-priate allergen. But why do common environmental antigens, innocuous to the vast majority of individuals, cause such mayhem and distress to the small but significant minority? What is the immunopathological process and how does it arise?

The immunopathology of allergic reactions is well established. In a nutshell, three cell types – the mast cell, the eosinophil and the basophil, and one antibody isotype – IgE – are central to the allergic reaction. Atopic individuals (those with a predisposition to allergic reactions) produce large amounts of allergen-specific IgE on exposure to an allergen. Mast cells (and basophils/eosinophils) express surface Fc receptors to which the Fc region of IgE can bind, so that after primary exposure to the allergen the cell surface has large numbers of IgE molecules. On subsequent exposure, the allergen can cross-link the IgE molecules on the mast cell surface, drag-ging the Fc receptors together, and thus leading to mast cell degranulation, with the release of granules containing histamine and other powerful vasoactive amines that then cause the typical symptoms (Figure 5.4).

Although the mast/eosinophil/basophil degranulation releases powerful chemi-cals that cause significant debility for the sufferer, these reactions are in fact normal and important in immunological responses, as they provide a defense against para-sites that are too large to be phagocytosed by macrophages and other professional phagocytes.

The vast majority of people do not suffer from allergies following exposure to the same antigens, their immune systems either ignoring the allergens altogether or

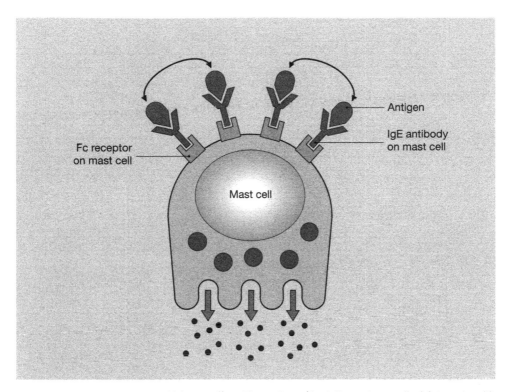

Figure 5.4 Type I hypersensitivity reaction. The antigen (the 'allergen', or pollen) interacts with immunoglobulin (IgE) bound to tissue mast cells, basophils or eosinophils. The cross-linking of IgE by the antigen results in membrane destabilization and release of granules containing histamine and other powerful vasoactive amines that cause the typical symptoms of asthma, rhinitis and conjunctivitis. Susceptible individuals are thought to have a genetic defect in antigen processing which results in synthesis of IgE rather than IgG in response to certain allergens such as grass pollen, house dust, etc.

responding weakly, producing mainly T_{h1} helper cells and low levels of IgG antibodies. So why do some individuals respond by producing IgE?

Type II hypersensitivity reactions

The obstetrician and gynecologist would not routinely come across patients with these types of immunological reactions, but they are described briefly here for completeness. Type II reactions are initiated by antibody reacting with antigenic determinants which form part of the cell membrane. The outcome of the reactions depends on whether or not complement or accessory cells become involved, and whether the metabolism of the cell is affected (Figure 5.5). As can be seen from Figure 5.5, type II hypersensitivity is the basis of a wide range of disease processes.

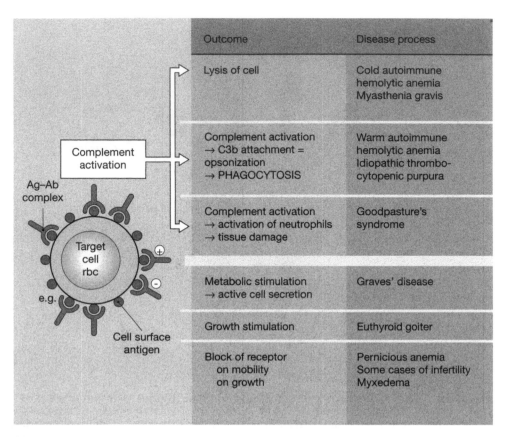

Figure 5.5 Type II hypersensitivity reaction. Ag, antigen; Ab, antibody; rbc, red blood cell

Type III hypersensitivity reactions

These reactions are caused by immune complexes in the circulation or in the tissues. Large quantities of immune complexes in the tissues may activate complement and accessory cells, thereby causing an inflammatory reaction with extensive tissue damage. The classic example is the so-called Arthus reaction, where an antigen is injected into the skin of an animal that has been previously sensitized. The pre-formed antibody reacts with the antigen, resulting in high concentrations of local immune complexes which activate complement, which in turn attracts neutrophils and results in local inflammation 6–24 h after injection. Clinical examples of this type of hypersensitivity include SLE (see above), glomerulonephritis, serum sickness and extrinsic allergic alveolitis. As the damaging complexes are formed, the antigen concentration is rapidly lowered. The process continues only as long as the antigen persists, and thus is usually self-limiting (Figure 5.6).

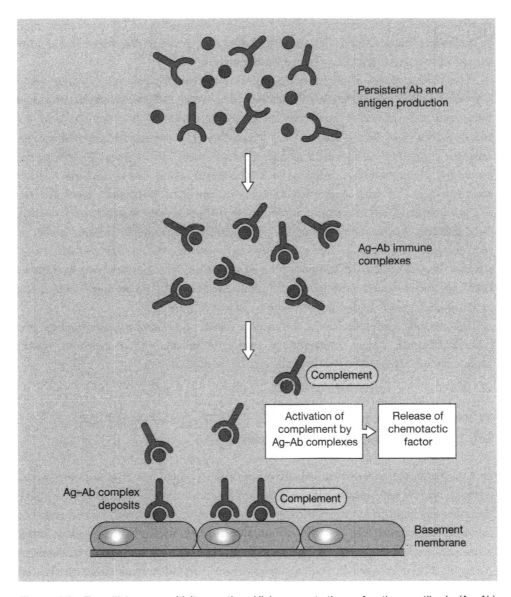

Figure 5.6 Type III hypersensitivity reaction. High concentrations of antigen–antibody (Ag–Ab) immune complexes due to persistent antigen and antibody production lead to complement activation and inflammation with extensive tissue damage. Clinical examples are: systemic lupus erythematosus, serum sickness, some glomerulonephritis, extrinsic allergic alveolitis

Type IV or delayed hypersensitivity

Although tuberculosis (TB) is most commonly perceived as an infection involving the lungs, the gynecologist will be familiar with tuberculous endometritis, resulting in amenorrhea and/or infertility. This is common in areas where TB is endemic, such as the Indian subcontinent. The basic pathological processes that occur in the lung are similar to those that occur in the endometrium.

The TB bacterium invading the endometrium is engulfed by macrophages, playing their normal role in defense of the body. In normal circumstances, the engulfed bacterium is destroyed by powerful chemicals contained in lysosomes within the macrophages. Alas, in the case of TB, the bacterium resists destruction and escapes into the cytoplasm of the macrophage where it multiplies, eventually killing the macrophage and further escaping into the surrounding tissue to infect other macrophages. The dead macrophage releases its powerful lysosomal chemicals into the surrounding endometrium, initiating an inflammatory reaction and causing local damage. Additional cytokines are produced that increase the 'killing' power of macrophages, and also attract other immune-system cells to the endometrium, thereby increasing the inflammatory response. When the immune system fails to eradicate the invaders, chronic inflammation ensues, with the endometrium being gradually destroyed by the inflammatory reaction (Figure 5.7).

Tuberculous endometritis is a common cause of secondary amenorrhea and infertility in the Indian subcontinent, and an example of the immune system mounting a normal response, but culminating in disease.

SUPERANTIGENS AND THE EXCESSIVE STIMULATION OF T CELLS AND MACROPHAGES

In Chapter 1, the basis of the adaptive immune response was that a conventional protein antigen activates only those T lymphocytes that bear a TcR specific for peptides derived from the antigen, which are a tiny subset of the total T cell pool. For example, only about one in 10 000 circulating T cells from donors immunized with tetanus toxoid subsequently proliferates when stimulated by the toxoid. In contrast, a special class of antigens known as superantigens directly activate large numbers of T cells carrying a particular TcR Vβ gene. In contrast to conventional antigens which are processed intracellularly before being presented within an MHC peptide groove to the TcR, superantigens simultaneously bind as the whole unprocessed protein to MHC class II molecules outside the peptide-binding groove and also to the lateral face of certain subsets of Vβ chains of the TcR (Figure 5.8).

Superantigens are bacterial and viral proteins which cross-link MHC class II molecules and TcRs, resulting in the activation of both the T cell and the APC as a result of signals initiated by the TcR and the MHC molecule, respectively. Each superantigen is capable of binding to a limited group of Vβ regions. The toxic shock

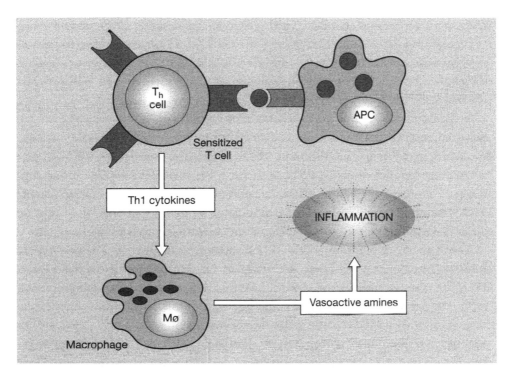

Figure 5.7 Type IV hypersensitivity reaction. T cells react with antigen and release helper T cell (Th1) cytokines, which attract other cells, particularly macrophages, which in turn liberate lysosomal enzymes. A chronic inflammatory reaction ensues with consequent tissue damage. Clinical examples are: tuberculosis, tuberculoid leprosy, contact dermatitis, graft rejection, graft-versus-host disease. APC, antigen-presenting cell

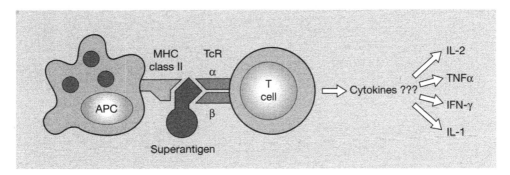

Figure 5.8 Superantigen-induced T cell stimulation. Superantigens interact with T cell receptors (TcRs) and major histocompatibility complex (MHC) class II molecules in a way distinct from the way that normal peptide antigens bind. Superantigens are not processed by the antigen-presenting cell (APC), but bind independently as a whole protein antigen to the Vb domain of the TcR and the MHC class II, away from the peptide-binding site. Large amounts of cytokines are produced which mediate the clinical picture. IL, interleukin; TNF, tumor necrosis factor; IFN, interferon

syndrome is an example familiar to gynecologists. The toxic shock syndrome toxin-1 (TSST-1), which is produced by certain strains of the Gram-positive bacterium *Staphylococcus aureus*, stimulates all those T cells that express the Vβ2 gene segment. As there is a limited repertoire of Vβ gene segments, any superantigen will stimulate between 2 and 20% of all T cells.

It is important to note that the mode of stimulation is not specific for the pathogen, and thus does not lead to adaptive immunity. Instead, it causes excessive production of cytokines (interleukin-1 (IL-1), TNF, IL-2, interferon-γ (IFN-γ), etc.) by the large number of activated CD4 T cells, the predominant responding population. The massive cytokine release causes systemic toxicity (manifesting as toxic shock syndrome), and suppression of the adaptive immune response, both of these effects contributing to the pathogenicity of microbes that produce superantigens.

The toxic shock syndrome (TSS) is known to gynecologists as a serious disease characteristically occurring in menstruating women, typically in their teenage years, but in fact cases occur in all age groups. It is usually associated with a tampon being left in the vagina for more than 12 h where, soaked in menstrual fluids, it enhances the growth of the bacteria that produce the superantigen TSST-1. TSS presents with rapid onset of fever, a rash, organ failure and shock, and unless dealt with appropriately it can be fatal. Immediate management includes admission to intensive care and cardiovascular support with intravenous fluid, and once all specimens have been taken, the commencement of appropriate broad-spectrum antibiotics intravenously. Any tampon in the vagina should be removed. Often the diagnosis is not immediately apparent until the patient has been stabilized and already making a recovery.

Apart from TSS, superantigens are thought to play a role in staphylococcal food poisoning, streptococcal TSS, scarlet fever, HIV and rabies, to name but a few.

6

Immunological tests in obstetrics and gynecology

It is sometimes easy to forget that many of the tests routinely and frequently used in both obstetrics and gynecology have an immunological basis. The ubiquitous pregnancy test, for example, now so sensitive that the woman desperate to conceive can tell whether or not she is pregnant even before she misses her period, is basically an antibody and antigen interaction (Figure 6.1). Tests for immunity to rubella, or previous exposure to a whole host of other viruses, are all based on immunological principles. In this chapter, common tests that have an immunological basis are described. Central to most modern tests, especially the sensitivity and specificity, is the monoclonal antibody. Before the advent of monoclonal antibodies, antisera for diagnostic purposes were usually raised in animals by injection of the relevant antigen, i.e. the animals were immunized with the relevant antigen (for example β-human chorionic gonadotropin (hCG)). The animals responded by making polyclonal antibodies – the resultant sera contained mixtures of antibodies from different B cell clones. Although these antibodies varied in the precise nature of their variable regions, they all reacted only with epitopes on the relevant antigen (monospecific reactivity). Because the antisera contained a whole host of other proteins, before use for diagnostic purposes the polyclonal antibodies would be purified by eluting them on special columns under pH conditions that allowed initial binding of antibody to antigenic epitopes, and subsequent separation when the pH and other conditions were changed.

MONOCLONAL ANTIBODIES: THE ADVENT OF HYBRIDOMA TECHNOLOGY

The technique of producing monoclonal antibodies by somatic cell hybridization was first described by Georges J. F. Kohler and César Milstein in 1975. This

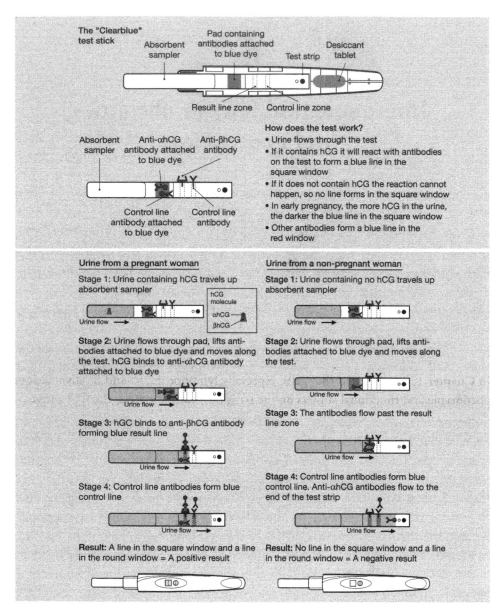

Figure 6.1 Immunological basis of the pregnancy test. Any woman suspecting that she might be pregnant no longer needs the services of a doctor. The pregnancy test kits now available in any high street pharmacy allow the woman to conduct a pregnancy test in the privacy of her home, with accuracy in excess of 99%. The kits generally work by the detection of the pregnancy hormone human chorionic gonadotropin (hCG) present in the urine of pregnant women, and the underlying principle is based on an antigen–antibody reaction. The 'Clearblue' test stick is used as an example to illustrate how the pregnancy test works. The test is a sandwich immunoassay employing monoclonal antibodies specific to hCG and uses chromatographic principles to separate bound and free colored label. The kit incorporates two indicators – a control line which shows that the test has worked correctly, and the test result line, the two appearing in two different windows. Courtesy of Unipath Ltd.

technique has been employed by immunologists to prepare virtually unlimited quantities of antibodies that are chemically, physically and immunologically completely homogeneous. When the extent of their use in both clinical diagnosis and research is considered, it is almost impossible to understand how it was ever possible to manage without them. Such was the significance of this discovery that Kohler and Milstein were awarded the Nobel Prize for Immunology in 1984. A curious but true *faux pas* in this story is that Kohler and Milstein overlooked patenting their discovery prior to publication of the details of their technique, thus depriving themselves and their institute of a fortune in royalties!

The principle underpinning hybridoma technology is fundamentally simple: a plasma cell (which by definition produces an antibody of a single specificity, see Chapter 1) is fused with a non-secreting myeloma cell line to form a 'hybridoma', which has the antibody-producing capacity of the parent B cell and the immortality of the malignant plasma cell. The detail is described in Figure 6.2.

FLOW CYTOMETRY

In Chapter 1, it was stated that cells, especially lymphocytes, could be divided into phenotypic and functional subsets on the basis of surface markers, the CD antigens. These markers are of course identified by the monoclonal antibodies produced by the hybridoma technology described above. Although over the years there has been a plethora of techniques for analyzing and separating lymphocyte cell subsets, flow cytometry has emerged as the most discriminating procedure for analysis and sorting of cells based on their surface markers. The principles on which flow cytometry work are described in Figure 6.3. Quantitation of T and B lymphocyte subpopulations is essential in immunodeficiency and useful in lymphoproliferative disease. The number of circulating CD4 positive T lymphocytes is a strong prognostic factor in human immunodeficiency virus (HIV) infection (Chapter 5), and is used as a surrogate marker for assessing progress of the disease and the need for, and response to, anti-HIV therapy. Flow cytometry has recently been used to study natural killer (NK) cell populations and activity in women with recurrent spontaneous miscarriage. Flow cytometry has also been used to search for fetal cells in the maternal circulation: a potentially non-invasive prenatal diagnosis which was embraced with the promise of replacing chorionic villus sampling and amniocentesis, but has failed to deliver, probably because the occurrence of fetal cells in the maternal circulation is not a regular or consistent phenomenon. Outside obstetrics and gynecology there is of course a wide application of flow cytometry.

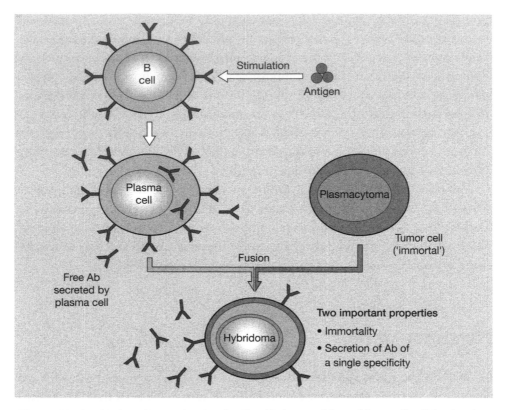

Figure 6.2 Production of monoclonal antibodies. Under special conditions, a B cell that has been stimulated by its specific antigen (Ag) can be fused with a plasmacytoma to produce a hybridoma, which is 'immortal' and can produce unlimited quantities of an antibody (Ab) of a single specificity

Although they are complex devices, flow cytometers in fact work on relatively simple principles (Figure 6.3). The flow cytometer is an optical/electronic device which measures cell size and can detect the presence of cell-bound fluorochrome-conjugated antibody. A single-cell suspension containing the lymphocytes of interest labeled with fluorochrome-conjugated antibody is forced through the nozzle of the device, under pressure. The cells are confined to the axis of the resultant fluid stream by a concentric sheath of cell-free fluid. A laser beam is focused onto the stream and two important events occur: the light excites the cell membrane-bound fluorochromes; and the light itself is scattered and reflected by the cells. The light emitted by the excited fluorochromes, and that scattered and reflected by the cells, is detected by a suitable arrangement of lenses, optical filters and photoelectric devices. The electrical signals generated are analyzed by computer, and are also used to activate the cell-sorting process. Sorting depends on breaking up the fluid stream and electrically charging the droplets, so that for instance the droplets containing

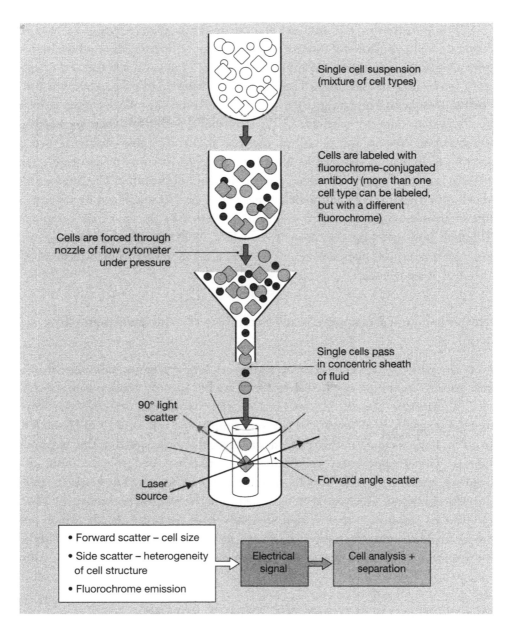

Figure 6.3 Principles of flow cytometry

brightly fluorescent cells may be given a positive charge, and those containing dull cells a negative one. Positively charged drops are deflected to a negative plate where they are collected into sterile tissue culture medium, while the negatively charged drops are deflected to a positive plate and discarded.

Cell populations vary in size and granularity. These properties can be used to define the cell population of interest in a suspension of mixed cells or whole blood, prior to analysis by monoclonal antibodies. Specified limits on cell size and granularity can be used to 'gate' the cell population, ensuring that further analysis is confined to these cells. The data are then displayed as a series of profile histograms, with the fluorescent intensity generated by the monoclonal antibody shown on the horizontal axis and the number of cells on the vertical axis. If double labeling is used, a dot plot of individual cells can be obtained, where the intensity of fluorescence of one dye is plotted against the intensity of fluorescence of the other. The proportions of cells reactive with both antibodies, either one or neither are shown by the intensity of the dots, and quantitative results are generated by the machine's computer. Although flow cytometers are expensive to buy, results are obtained quickly and easily by experienced users, and results are very accurate owing to the vast numbers of cells that are counted.

Antibody-coupled magnetic beads as cell sorters: the 'poor man's flow cytometer'

As an alternative to flow cytometry for sorting cell subpopulations, monoclonal antibody-labeled immunomagnetic beads can be used to identify and separate cell subsets. While there are several variations on the theme, the principle on which immunomagnetic beads work is in fact very simple, and is illustrated in Figure 6.4. In essence, monoclonal antibody of a desired specificity is coupled to tiny magnetic spheres. Under appropriate conditions the antibody-coated spheres (immunomagnetic beads) are incubated with the cell mixture of interest. The beads attach to the cells of interest, which are then separated from the mixture on a magnetic plate. Innovations resulting from magnetic beads have included beads which are biodegradable, so that the separated cells can be included in an experiment without the need to take the extra step to separate out the beads!

DETECTION OF AUTOANTIBODIES IN SERUM

Four standard methods are commonly used in the detection of circulating autoantibodies: immunofluorescence, particle agglutination, immunoassay and counter current electrophoresis. Each type of assay system has its own advantages and disadvantages. Immunofluorescence is the least sensitive of these techniques, and depends on subjective interpretation by an experienced observer. Particle agglutination is more sensitive but more time-consuming. Radioimmunoassays (RIAs) require

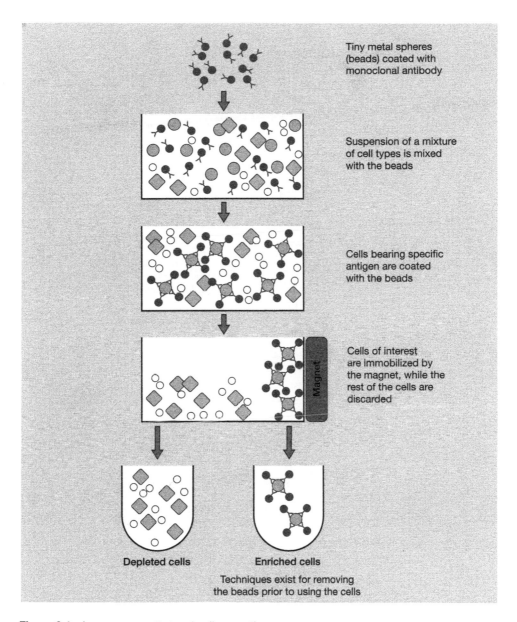

Tiny metal spheres (beads) coated with monoclonal antibody

Suspension of a mixture of cell types is mixed with the beads

Cells bearing specific antigen are coated with the beads

Cells of interest are immobilized by the magnet, while the rest of the cells are discarded

Depleted cells   Enriched cells

Techniques exist for removing the beads prior to using the cells

Figure 6.4 Immunomagnetic bead cell separation

expensive reagents, facilities for γ and β counting of radioisotopes and appropriate facilities for handling and disposal of radioactive waste. Enzyme-linked immunosorbent assays (ELISAs) avoid the problems of radioisotope handling and disposal, but also require specialized equipment. Counter current electrophoresis is easy and cheap, but relatively insensitive.

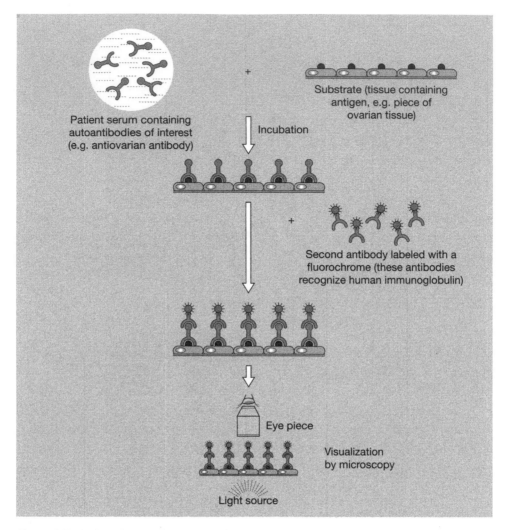

Figure 6.5 Indirect immunofluorescence for the detection of autoantibodies in serum

Indirect immunofluorescence

Tissues known to express the putative antigen are snap-frozen and sections are cut at −20°C on cryostat. The patient's serum is incubated with the tissue sections (substrate) for 30 min, and the unbound proteins are then washed off before a second antibody, with a visible tag (usually fluorescein), is added. This reacts with those serum immunoglobulins which have combined with antigens in the substrate. The site of antibody fixation can then be visualized by fluorescent microscopy (Figure 6.5).

Where relevant, a positive serum is titrated to determine the strength of the antibody. The results are expressed as a titer or in international units if a known standard has been used for comparison. Several autoantibodies can be detected simultaneously by using a composite block of tissue. Interpretation of the results depends on the class and titer of the antibody and the age and sex of the patient. The elderly, especially women, are prone to develop autoantibodies in the absence of clinical autoimmune disease. In contrast, high-titer autoantibodies in a child or young adult suggest that overt disease may appear later. The antinuclear antibody (ANA) test is an example of a test which is sensitive but not specific. The mere presence of ANA does not equate with autoimmune disease, and certainly not with systemic lupus erythematosus (SLE), but, by using an appropriate cut-off point, a negative ANA is strong screening evidence against the diagnosis. Over 95% of patients with SLE will be ANA-positive, but the false-positive rate will also be about 5–15%.

Particle agglutination

Particles of latex or gelatine or red blood cells are used as indicator particles which clump together when an antibody cross-links the antigens on their surfaces. The antigens may be native to the red cells (such as the ABO or other blood group antigens) or purified non-red cell antigens which have been coupled onto the particle or red cell surface. The use of agglutination depends on the availability of purified antigens. The method of coupling is irrelevant except in rheumatoid factor tests.

Rheumatoid factor (an immunoglobulin M (IgM) antibody which reacts with IgG as the antigen) reacts more strongly with aggregated IgG than with native human IgG. IgG is, therefore, aggregated by prior reaction with its given antigen (sheep red blood cells) or by heat. Most laboratories use a latex test for rheumatoid factor; heat-aggregated human IgG is attached to the latex particles, which agglutinate in the presence of rheumatoid factor. This is a quick and cheap test but gives a large number of false positives. The red cell agglutination test (Rose–Waller test) is more specific, but more expensive and time-consuming.

Radioimmunoassay (RIA) and enzyme-linked immunosorbent assay (ELISA)

These are extremely sensitive methods of detecting autoantibodies in low concentration. The same techniques are used in other branches of pathology, for example for hormonal assays (Figures 6.6 and 6.7). ELISAs are more sensitive but less specific than RIAs. Because the problem of handling and disposal of radioisotopes is

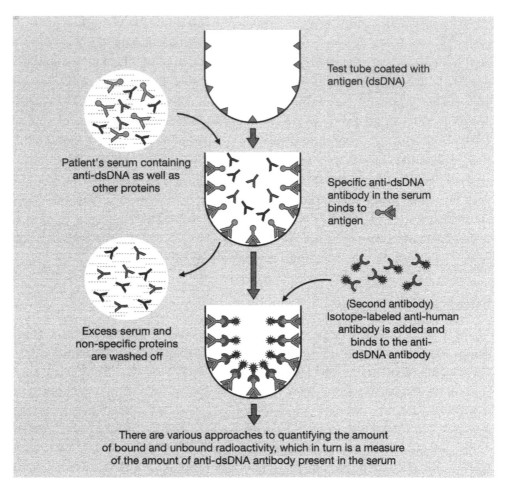

Figure 6.6 Principles of radioimmunoassay (RIA). The technique of RIA has revolutionized research and clinical practice in many areas including endocrinology, immunodiagnostics and blood banking to name but just three areas. RIA was introduced in 1960 as an assay for measuring the concentration of insulin in plasma. It represented the first time that hormone levels *in the blood* could be detected by an *in vitro* assay. RIA is widely used because of its great sensitivity. Using antibodies of high affinity it is possible to detect a few picograms (10^{-12} g) of antigen. The detection of an autoantibody, such as antibodies to double-stranded DNA (dsDNA) which occur in systemic lupus erythematosis (SLE) can be used to describe the underlying principle as shown here

avoided, the 'green' credentials mean that ELISAs are more commonly used in immunoassays.

Functional tests

In vitro tests of lymphocyte function should be performed only if the clinical features suggest abnormal cell-mediated immunity. These assays are, therefore, only essential in suspected T cell immunodeficiencies. These tests can be done using either whole

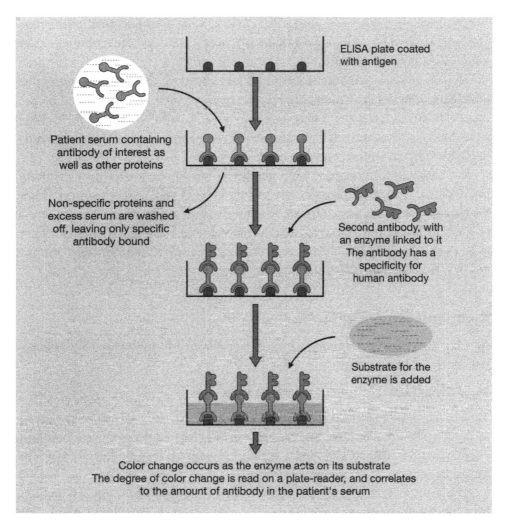

Figure 6.7 Principles of enzyme-linked immunosorbent assay (ELISA). ELISA tests are generally highly sensitive and specific and compare favorably with radioimmunoassay (RIA) tests. However, ELISAs have the added advantages of not needing radioisotopes or a radiation-counting apparatus, thus rendering them cheaper, safer and less cumbersome. While there are variations of the ELISA, the underlying principle is simple and can be described as shown here (note the similarity with RIA, except that the radioisotope is replaced by an enzyme)

blood or separated lymphocytes. Either way, fresh anticoagulated blood is required as viable cells are tested. Purification of lymphocytes from whole blood is achieved by layering heparinized blood onto a density gradient. On centrifugation, the red cells and polymorphs sink through the gradient, leaving lymphocytes and a few contaminating monocytes in an easily distinguishable band on the top of the gradient; the band is aspirated and the cells are washed.

When lymphocytes are activated by certain substances, a few small resting lymphocytes respond by changing into blast cells over a few days. This process is called lymphocyte transformation.

The proliferative response is measured by radioactive thymidine incorporation into DNA or by the expression of cell surface markers, such as CD69, found on activated cells after a few hours. These tests require tissue culture facilities and are time-consuming and expensive. The batch variability and lack of standards makes interpretation difficult without rigorous controls.

It is possible to measure a large number of soluble or intracellular cytokines, interleukins, surface adhesion molecules or receptors and their messenger RNAs. Such assays are readily available and non-invasive but, as yet, must be considered as research investigations, not as assays of proven clinical value in any disorder. However, they will undoubtedly find their way into routine clinical practice, and it is worth introducing the principles here (see Figure 6.8).

Assessment of neutrophils and monocytes

Absolute numbers of these cells can easily be calculated from the total and differential white cell blood counts.

Functional tests

Tests of neutrophil function are essential in patients with recurrent or severe staphylococcal or fungal infections. Neutrophils can be separated from whole blood using a sedimentation method and their functional property is broken down into a series of key steps.

The surface proteins which mediate adhesion of neutrophils to vascular endothelium are the β2 family. The proteins have a common β chain (CD18) which combines with different α chains (CD11a, CD11b and CD11c) to form heterodimers including leukocyte function antigen 1 (LFA-1: CD11a/CD18) and complement receptor 3 (CR3: CD11b/CD18). In leukocyte adhesion deficiency, there is a genetic defect of CD18 with non-functional receptors preventing normal neutrophil adhesion to vascular endothelium. These markers are variably expressed on neutrophils, although detection of CD18 is reliable, and thus absence of this marker is significant.

Chemotaxis is the purposeful movement of cells toward an attractant, usually casein, or a synthetic peptide. The ability of the patient's serum to generate chemotactic effectors can be tested by incubating fresh serum with toxin. In the leading-front type of assay, the cells to be tested are separated from the chemotactic stimulus by a millipore membrane. After incubation, the filter membrane is removed,

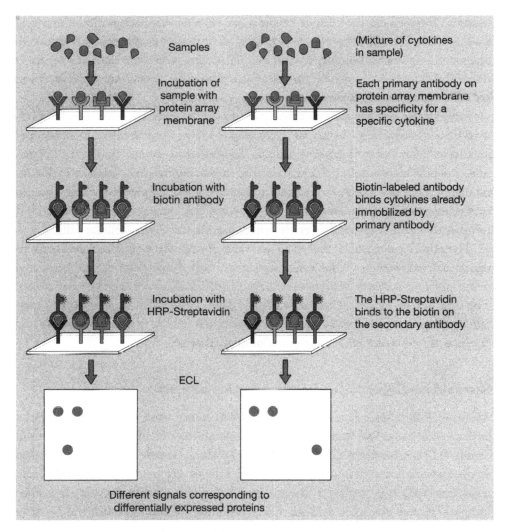

Figure 6.8 Protein array technology. It has become apparent in recent years that cytokines play a central role in reproduction (see Chapter 2 for examples of Th1 and Th2 cytokines). However, it is also clear that the measurement of a single cytokine in isolation is unlikely to provide a dynamic picture of the role of individual cytokines. Protein array technology allows simultaneous detection of multiple cytokines in one hybridization experiment. This technology is applicable to a wide range of proteins to which an antibody can be raised, since in essence the principle of antigen–antibody interaction is central to the technology. The basic principle on which this technology works is illustrated here

fixed and stained. The distance that cells have migrated through the filter towards the stimulus can be measured using a conventional light microscope. Chemotaxis is not used routinely, but can be helpful as a research assay.

Phagocytosis is the ingestion of foreign material. Ingestion can be determined by incubation of phagocytic cells with inert particles, such as latex beads, or yeasts or bacteria. Intracellular particles or bacteria can be seen microscopically. Cross-over studies using normal controls allow testing of a patient's cells for the ability to phagocytose particles opsonized with normal serum, while the patient's serum is tested for its ability to opsonize particles for ingestion by normal neutrophils. These are still predominantly research assays.

Intracellular enzyme activity accompanying the 'respiratory burst' can be measured by bacterial killing. A standard intracellular killing assay involves incubation of leukocytes with viable organisms, such as *Staphylococcus aureus*. Following incubation, the cells are washed and centrifuged to remove extracellular organisms. Bacteria ingested but not killed are then cultured by lysing the cells with distilled water to release ingested bacteria onto nutrient. Provided that phagocytosis is normal, the number of viable organisms inversely reflects the degree of intracellular killing.

The nitro blue tetrazolium (NBT) test measures the ability of phagocytic cells to ingest and reduce this soluble yellow dye to an intracellular blue crystal. Separated neutrophils are added to a solution containing NBT and stimulated with endotoxin. The cells can be viewed microscopically to count the number of polymorphs containing blue crystals. This is an easy screening test which is widely available and essential for exclusion of chronic granulomatous disease.

Recombinant DNA technology and cutting-edge tests

Although this chapter is mainly concerned with tests whose underlying principles have an immunological basis, it would be remiss not to include brief descriptions of tests based on recombinant DNA technology which are closely linked and often used in close conjuction with immunological tests. One of the fundamental principles in molecular pathology testing is the use of DNA probes, which are simply known unique segments of nucleic acid sequences which can be used to detect the presence or otherwise of complementary sequences of DNA (or RNA) in patient samples. The probe is a single strand of DNA, and its reactivity with its complementary target in a mixture of large amounts of nucleotide bases is called *DNA hybridization*, which is the most specific intermolecular interaction known between biological macromolecules.

The polymerase chain reaction (PCR)

PCR is an *in vitro* method for the selective and rapid amplification of as little as a single molecule of DNA into millions of billions of copies. The principles of PCR are illustrated in Figure 6.9. Briefly, PCR uses enzymes to amplify a chosen DNA molecule. The two coiled strands of DNA are uncoiled into single strands by heating

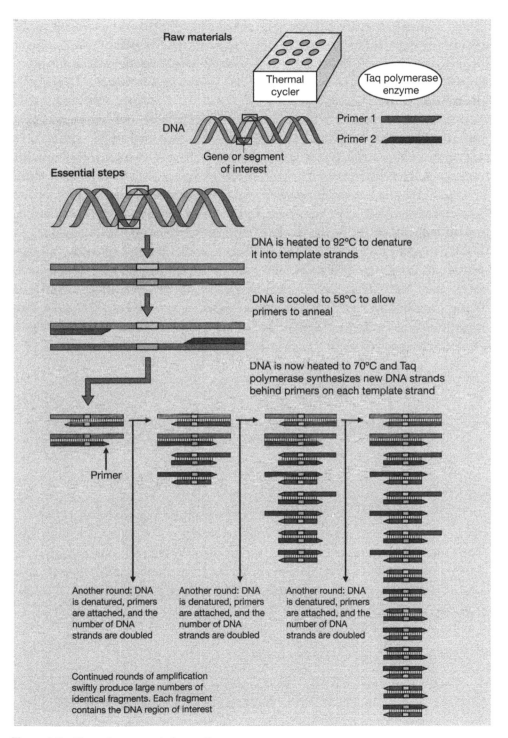

Figure 6.9 The polymerase chain reaction

at high temperature (92ºC). Two short strands, the primers, are hybridized to the strands on either side of the target DNA fragment (the template). A thermostable bacterial enzyme (derived from the bacterium *Thermus aquaticus* which thrives in hot springs – hence the enzyme is called Taq polymerase for short), a DNA polymerase that synthesizes a new DNA strand, is added. The enzyme can only extend existing single strands of DNA, and so make new DNA only over the target region. After the first cycle of synthesis, there are now four strands of DNA in place of the original two. These strands form double helices which can be uncoiled again, so that primers can be hybridized and the whole process of synthesis of new DNA repeated, each cycle essentially doubling the amount of DNA fragment produced in the previous cycle, since each new strand can act as a template. This exponential production of large amounts of a specific DNA fragment can produce useful quantities of DNA in a matter of hours. PCR can be used to amplify a single molecule of target sequence in a complex mixture of DNA or RNA, and will amplify a single-copy gene in genomic DNA. It has played a vital role in the discovery of the gene for cystic fibrosis, for example, and in popular media people are probably more familiar with its use in forensics, trapping criminals on the basis of a single strand of hair or a single spermatozoon recovered from the scene of crime.

Index

T - #0615 - 071024 - C0 - 246/189/9 - PB - 9780367391232 - Gloss Lamination